Anne Rothstein
Scholar
Herbert H. Lehman College, CUNY

Linda Catelli
Elementary Consultant
Queens College, CUNY

Patt Dodds
Instructional Designer
University of Massachusetts

Joan Manahan
Secondary Consultant
Teaneck, New Jersey

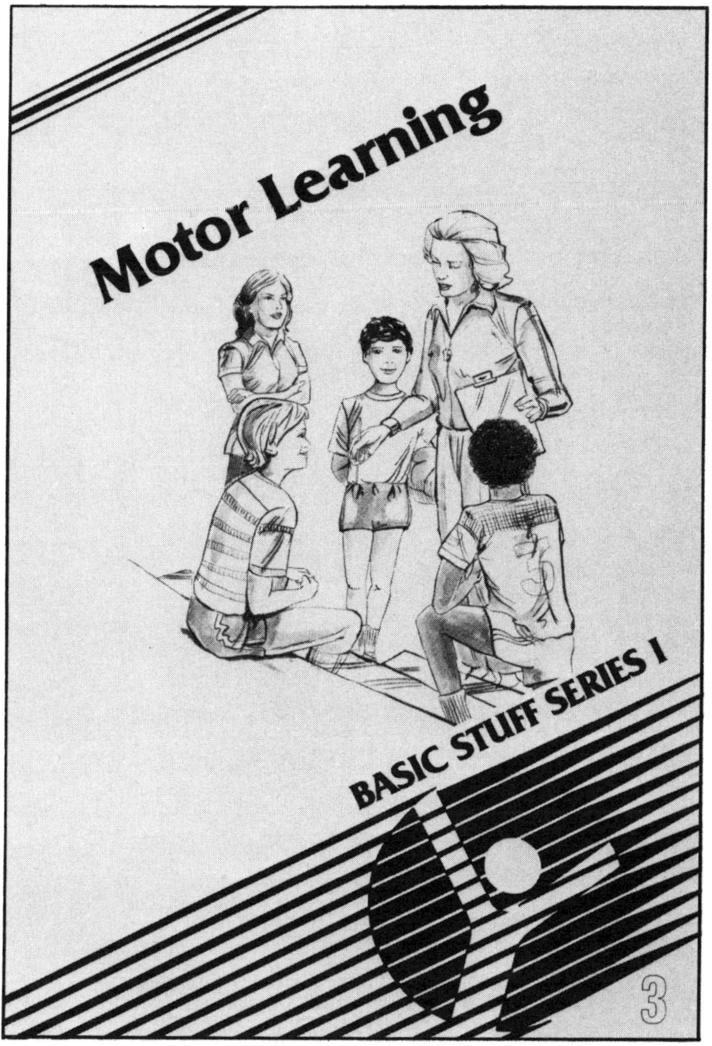

American Alliance for Health,
Physical Education, Recreation and Dance
1900 Association Drive, Reston, VA 22091

ISBN 0-88314-026-8

A Project of the
National Association for Sport and Physical Education
An Association of the
American Alliance for Health, Physical Education,
Recreation and Dance

"BASIC STUFF" SERIES

A collection of booklets presenting the body of knowledge in physical education and sport for practitioners and students.

"BASIC STUFF" SERIES

Series One **Informational Booklets**

- **Exercise Physiology**
- **Kinesiology**
- **Motor Learning**
- **Psycho-Social Aspects of Physical Education**
- **Humanities in Physical Education**
- **Motor Development**

Series Two **Learning Experience Booklets**

- **Early Childhood**
- **Childhood**
- **Adolescence**

preface

The information explosion has hit physical education. Researchers are discovering new links between exercise and human physiology. Others are investigating neurological aspects of motor control. Using computer simulation and other sophisticated techniques, biomechanics researchers are finding new ways to analyze human movement. As a result of renewed interest in social, cultural, and psychological aspects of movement, a vast, highly specialized body of knowledge has emerged.

Many physical education teachers want to use and apply information particularly relevant to their teaching. It is not an easy task. The quantity of research alone would require a dawn to dusk reading schedule. The specialized nature of the research tends to make it difficult for a layperson to comprehend fully. And finally, little work has been directed toward applying the research to the more practical concerns of teachers in the field. Thus the burgeoning body of information available to researchers and academicians has had little impact on physical education programs in the field.

The Basic Stuff series is the culmination of the National Association for Sport and Physical Education efforts to confront this problem. An attempt was made to identify basic knowledge relevant to physical education programs and to present that knowledge in a useful, readable format. The series is not concerned with physical education curriculum design, but the "basic stuff" concepts are common core information pervading any physical education course of study.

The selection of knowledge for inclusion in the series was based upon its relevance to students in physical education programs. Several common student motives or purposes for participation were identified: health (feeling good), appearance (looking good), achievement (doing better), social (getting along), aesthetic (turning on), and coping with the environment (surviving). Concepts were then selected which provided information useful to students in accomplishing these purposes.

The Basic Stuff project includes two types of booklets. Series I is designed for use by preservice and inservice teachers and consists of six pamphlets concerning disciplinary areas: exercise physiology, kinesiology, motor development and motor learning, social/psychological aspects of movement, and movement in the humanities (art, history, philosophy). This first series summarizes information on student purposes. Series II is also designed for use by teachers but with a different focus. Three handbooks are included: early childhood; childhood; adolescence. Each describes examples of instructional activities which could be used to teach appropriate physical education concepts to each age group.

The development of the Basic Stuff series has been a cooperative effort of teams of scholars and public school teachers. Scholars provided the expertise in the content areas and in the development of instructional materials. Public school teachers identified relevance to students, field tested instructional activities, and encouraged the scholars to write for general understanding.

The format of the booklets was designed to be fun and readable. Series I is structured as a question and answer dialogue between students and a teacher. Series II continues this emphasis with the infusion of knowledge into the world of physical education instructional programs. Our hope is that the Basic Stuff series can help to make this scenario a reality.

Linda L. Bain, *Editorial Committee*
University of Houston

table of contents

foreword

Motor Learning has many assumed names: motor behavior, motor control, motor performance. Regardless of the label the goal is the same: exploration and explanation of the materials, methods, and mechanisms that underlie the learning and performance of motor skill. In keeping with this goal this book focuses on one of six questions suggested by the NASPE Editorial Board guiding this project, "What do you have to help me do better." While there is disagreement that doing better will help students *feel good, look good, get along, turn on,* and *survive,* these last five are more directly answered through concepts drawn from exercise physiology, biomechanics, social psychology, humanities and motor development.

In answering the question, *"What do you have to help me do better?,"* the book focuses on a different set of concepts which can be used to enhance student learning and performance throughout its eight chapters. Specific examples of how these concepts and ideas can be incorporated into learning and practice sessions are provided in this book as well as in the Series II books in this Basic Stuff series.

The chapters consider aspects of learning and performance such as: "What types of skills will I learn?" (Chapter Two), "Should I practice different skills in different ways?" (Chapter Four), "How can I have good timing?" (Chapter Six), and "How can I use feedback to improve performance?" (Chapter Seven). In addition Chapter Five provides suggestions for how performance might be evaluated to trace student improvement. Finally Chapter Eight summarizes the major changes that take place as learning occurs. This may provide an idea of what to expect as learning occurs or help to evaluate learning progress.

To make this booklet more readable, traditional methods of referencing have been avoided. Thus normal acknowledgement of the work and ideas of others via references to specific books or articles has been bypassed. However the sources used to write this manuscript should not go unacknowledged as I am indebted to many individual authors and researchers whose published work has contributed, generally or specifically, to this book. The material on skill types in Chapters Two and Four draws upon work done by A.M. Gentile, J. Higgins, R. Arnold, J. Billings, and M. Robb. The feedback chapter is influenced by the work of A.M. Gentile, P. DelRey, D. Holding, and G. Miller while the material on performance changes in learning comes from the work of R. Arnold, R.A. Schmidt, C. Bard, M. Fleury, R. Martenuik, and A.M. Gentile. The material on practice variables (Chapter Three) incorporates the work of R. Singer, G. Sage, and J. Oxendine. In incorporating the concepts and ideas of others I have tried to be consistent with their original intent. I take full responsibility for any distortion or errors which may have occurred.

Finally I would like to thank Patt Dodds and Joan Manahan for their assistance in this project. Special gratitude and thanks are due to Linda Catelli who worked tirelessly in seeing this project to completion and was invaluable in all phases. As the final common path through which all editorial suggestions and changes were funneled I must in the end be accountable to you, the reader, for any instances where this material misses its intended mark.

ALR
Newtown, Connecticut

August, 1980

CHAPTER ONE

achievement

SUCCESS

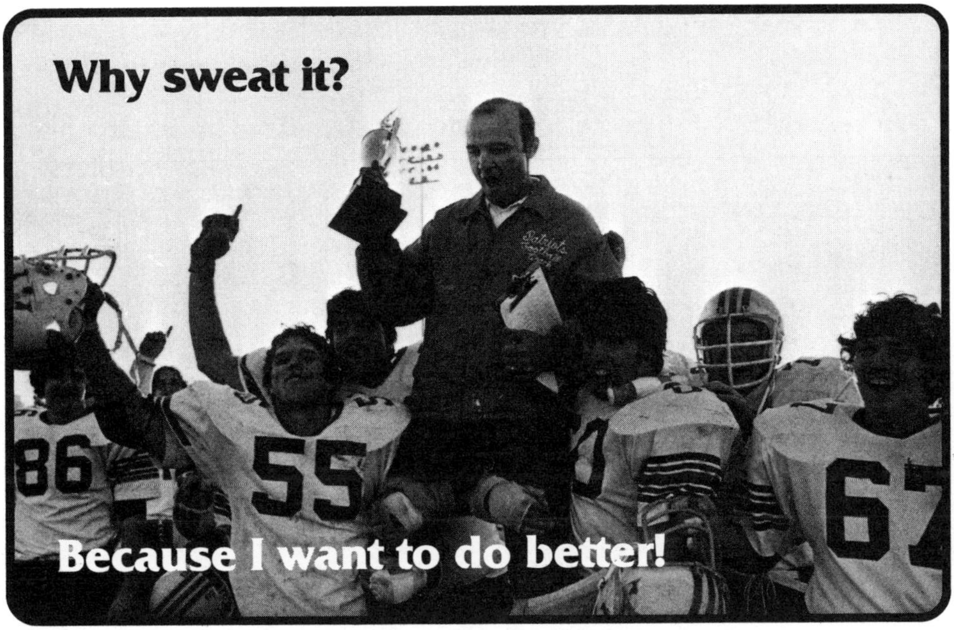

Photograph by Scott Forbes/Loudoun Times-Mirror

What Do You Have To Help Me?

The area of study called *motor learning* involves consideration of various factors which may affect learning and performance of skills used in sports and active games. One purpose of studying motor learning is to identify those factors which increase the likelihood of success at sports and active games. Most people want to be successful because it makes them feel good and it contributes to a positive self-image. One way to get this good feeling, to have this positive self-image, is to achieve set goals. Although individuals participate in a wide variety of activities, most devote some time to sports and active games. Motor learning can help contribute to success in sports and active games by identifying factors which are related to learning and performance. Therefore it can help people do better.

Motor learning can contribute to success in performing sports and games

Achieving success in motor skills performance requires effort and concentration. Individuals learning to perform motor skills sometimes waste their time and that of others because they don't know the most effective or efficient ways of learning motor skills. This book is intended to help students use learning and practice time to best advantage by sharing ideas concerning how they can learn motor skills faster and better. A way of organizing the discussion is by first identifying factors that individuals have to consider when learning or performing a skill and then discussing ways in which students might improve in each of these areas.

The information processing notion is a way of explaining the acquisition and performance of motor skills

It is helpful if the identified factors can be organized into an overall framework. A recent organizing framework used in describing motor learning and performance, which provides a good overall picture of the factors, involves the notion of information processing.

In order to be successful in performing motor skills the learner must be able to:

- pay attention to the right aspects of the environment (INPUT);
- select or plan a motor response which is compatible with the environment (DECISION-MAKING);
- execute the movement as planned (OUTPUT);
- utilize movement and outcome information to evaluate the present response and, if necessary, modify the next response (FEEDBACK).

It is not sufficient that each of these aspects is done correctly in isolation; the four operations must be integrated and must relate to each other so that control flows smoothly from one operation to another to conclude in successful performance. To become successful at performing skills, behavior must be adjusted within the four operations of INPUT, DECISION-MAKING, OUTPUT, and FEEDBACK. The role of feedback is unique because the learner not only improves in his ability to receive and use feedback; feedback is also absolutely necessary to improve the operation of the other processes.

Successful motor performance requires input, decision-making, output, and feedback

The relationship among the four operations which have been identified can be illustrated by a simple example. The performer 1) receives input, 2) makes a decision, 3) executes a response, and 4) receives feedback about movement execution and outcome. Let us suppose that you are playing in a basketball game and are in possession of the ball. First you obtain input about your position on the court, the position of your opponents and your teammates, and the distance between you and the basket. Second you analyze and interpret this information with reference to your past experience in the game of basketball and in situations similar to the present one and decide what type of response you will plan. The choice is based on information about your own past successes, past successes of your teammates in similar situations, and the options that are available to you. You decide whether to dribble, to pass to a teammate (including whom to pass to), to shoot from your present position (including what type of shot to take), or to stay put. You select one course of action and plan how to implement it.

Third, the movement planned is executed. Finally, during and after your response, FEEDBACK is received concerning the course of action taken. In assessing your movement you may ask such questions as: "Did I shoot the way I intended?," "Did I release the ball too early?," and "Did I follow through toward the basket?" After the response you receive FEEDBACK about the effect of your movement on the environment. In relation to the OUTCOME you ask such questions as: "Did I make the basket?" and "Was the pass accurate?"

How Do I Get It?

Can you identify examples of input, decision-making, output, and feedback?

Every skill you possess or will learn can be described in terms of the four major operations of INPUT, DECISION-MAKING, OUTPUT, and FEEDBACK. Some skills may involve one operation to a greater degree than other operations but all skills require all four. Using a familiar skill try to identify examples of input, decision-making, output, and feedback. In tennis, for example, some of the following may have been listed in each category:

INPUT
- ball direction
- ball speed
- ball spin
- opponent's position

DECISION-MAKING
- where ball will arrive (based on direction)
- when ball will arrive (based on speed)
- how ball will bounce (based on spin)
- select forehand, backhand, volley, etc.

OUTPUT
- when to initiate response
- actually performing the selected type

FEEDBACK

did I keep my wrist cocked? (MOVEMENT)
was my swing level? (MOVEMENT)
did I contact the ball in front of my forward foot? (MOVEMENT)
did the ball go over the net? (OUTCOME)
did the ball land in-bounds? (OUTCOME)
could my opponent hit the ball? (OUTCOME)

Information processing framework directs investigation of errors

Information processing can also be considered from the point of view of the unsuccessful performer. Knowing what must be accomplished to be successful can help us discern why someone is having difficulty in skill performance. For example did the individual make a mistake during the INPUT operation?, during the DECISION-MAKING operation?, during the OUTPUT operation?, during the FEEDBACK operation? That is did the individual look at the wrong place in the environment? (INPUT ERROR); did the individual misjudge the speed of the ball and/or its time of arrival? (DECISION-MAKING ERROR); did the person execute the movement faster than intended? (OUTPUT ERROR); did the individual fail to discriminate that the goal was not achieved, e.g., that the ball went out of bounds? (FEEDBACK ERROR). Additional examples of errors that can occur at each phase of information processing are presented in Table 1.1.

Why Does It Happen That Way?

Information processing explains behavior in terms of sequential operations

Information processing explains behavior in terms of a set of sequential operations that an individual performs to be successful at motor skills. These operations involve, in part:

- looking at the right place(s);
- paying attention to the right cue(s);
- interpreting what the cues signify;
- planning what to do (a response);
- organizing the response;
- doing the response;
- assessing how you moved and what effect it had.

These operations may be grouped into four categories:

INPUT

the processes involved in obtaining information;

DECISION-MAKING

analyzing and interpreting what the input means and deciding what to do about it;

Table 1.1: Examples of errors that might be made at the INPUT, DECISION-MAKING, OUTPUT, and FEEDBACK phases of information processing.

INPUT
- player looks at the wrong portion of the environment
- player pays attention to the wrong cues
- players attention is focused on too small an area
- players attention is focused on too broad an area
- player cannot see the relationship among the elements

DECISION-MAKING (interpretation of input)
- player misjudges the path, speed, or direction of teammate, object, or opponent
- player misjudges distances, heights, weights
- player miscalculates time of arrival of object, opponent, or teammate

DECISION-MAKING (selection of movement)
- player selects wrong type of movement
- player selects wrong instance of correct type of movement
- player misprograms time, force, direction, or distance of movement

OUTPUT
- player does not execute movement as planned

FEEDBACK
- player does not remember how he moved
- player cannot discriminate errors
- player cannot tell if goal was accomplished
- player cannot recognize what led to perceived error

OUTPUT

executing the response you decided on;

FEEDBACK

evaluating the performance (how you moved) and the outcome (the result).

The learner and the situation constitute a system

The individual who uses information processing to describe performance views the learner and the situation in which performance takes place as a *system*. This implies that the situation affects the performance and that the performance, in turn, affects the situation. Before giving an illustrative example of how this occurs it is helpful to know that *environment* is the term used to indicate the situation in which performance occurs. The *environment* includes both external and internal elements. The *external elements* of the environment at a basketball game may include, for each player:

- the positions of the other players;
- the distance to the basket;
- the location of the ball;
- the spectators;
- the score;
- the coach;
- the time remaining in the game.

Internal elements may include:

- fatigue;
- anxiety;
- pain;
- distracting thoughts.

Every situation in which sport takes place involves both internal and external elements. Some of the elements of the environment are important to success. Such things as the location of and distance to teammates, the location of and distance to opponents, and the distance to the basket are critical for successful performance. The spectators, feelings of anxiety, and distracting thoughts, may hamper performance if the player pays attention to them.

The situation affects the learner and the learner affects the situation

The learner and the environment should be considered a system. The environment affects behavior and behavior changes the environment. This affects subsequent behavior which further alters the environment. In a tennis match, for example, the position and speed of the ball dictates player A's position and swing; player A's hitting of the ball dictates player B's position and swing; player B's hitting of the ball in turn dictates player A's next position and swing and on and on until the rally is ended. The weave in basketball is an example of the interaction between a player and the environment

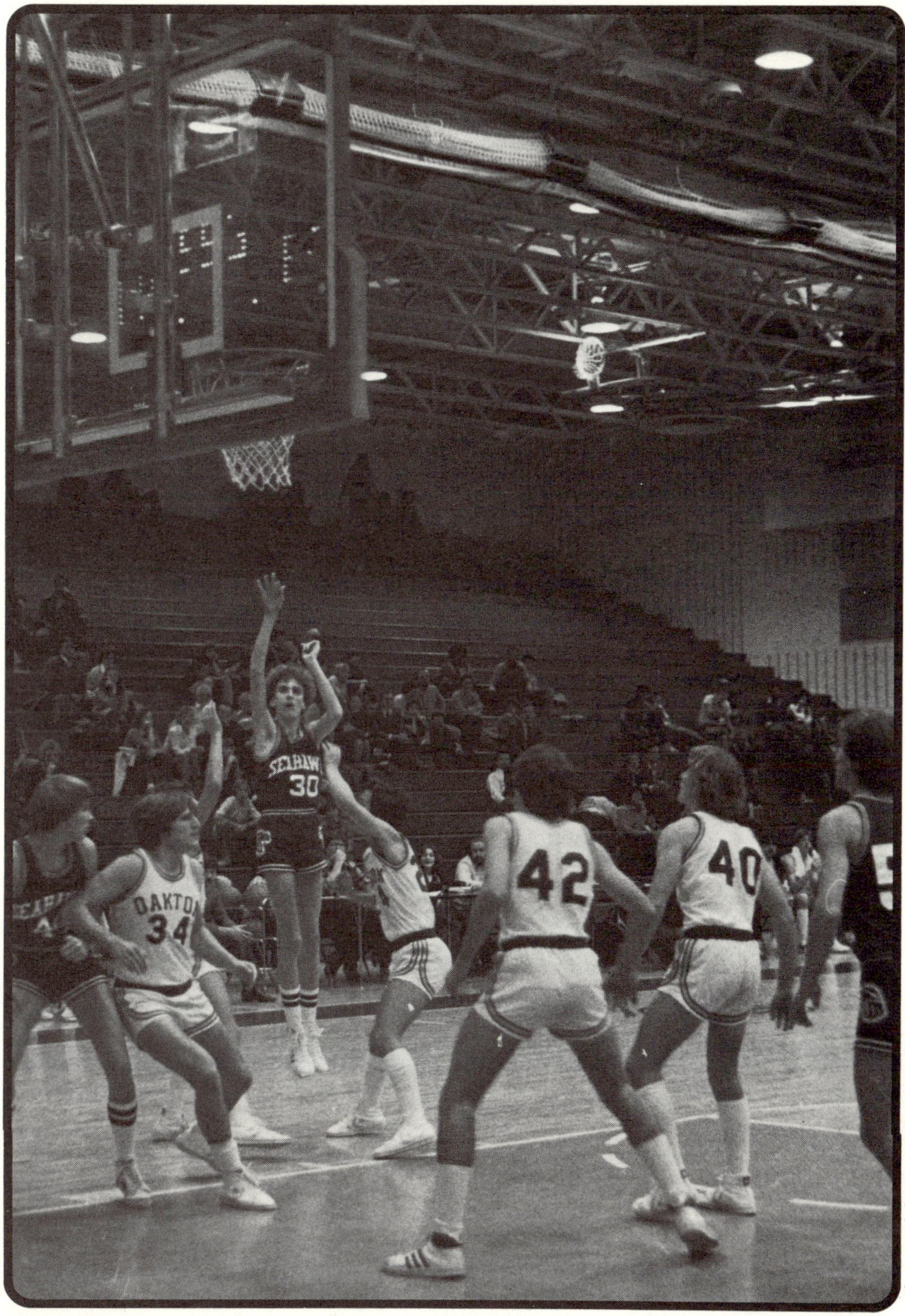

Photograph by Carlyjane Dunn Rice

External elements at a basketball game include the position of the other players, the distance to the basket, the location of the ball, and the spectators.

which, as we have seen, includes other players. As illustrated in Figure 1.1, player 1 passes to player 2 with the exact speed and direction of the pass depending on player 2's direction and speed of motion. Immediately upon executing the pass, player 1 has to respond to the altered environment by running behind player 2 to receive a pass from player 3 who has received the ball from player 2. Thus these three players form a small system in which the environment dictates the performance, the performance changes the environment, the new environment dictates the next performance and on and on until the basket is made or the opponents obtain the ball. Either of these last two possibilities changes the environment in ways that have special implications for performance and for the total system so that:

- a player interacts with the environment when executing a skill;
- the environment dictates how a player must move in order to be successful;
- a player's performance affects the environment by changing it in some way.

In summary the environment dictates when and how a player must move to be successful. Shooting a ball at a basket 10 feet away requires less force than shooting at a basket 20 feet away. If a receiver is running slow the ball does not have to be passed as far ahead as it would if a receiver is running fast.

Input is information from internal and external sources

As indicated earlier in this chapter *information processing* focuses on four major operations which affect sport performance: INPUT, DECISION-MAKING, OUTPUT, and FEEDBACK. INPUT is the label applied to all of the information in the environment that you *could* give attention when performing. Some of the INPUT will be important in relation to successful performances; other information will not be important at all. The input includes information from inside (internal) and outside (external) the body and is concerned about such aspects as:

- searching (looking for) and orienting (looking at) the right elements or cues;
- selective attention (concentrating on the critical cues and ignoring the non-critical cues);
- noise (the unnecessary information or non-critical cues which might be distracting).

These and other aspects of input will be considered in an effort to identify ways of learning new skills faster or improving present performance more quickly.

Figure 1.1: The player-environment system: a three-person weave in basketball.

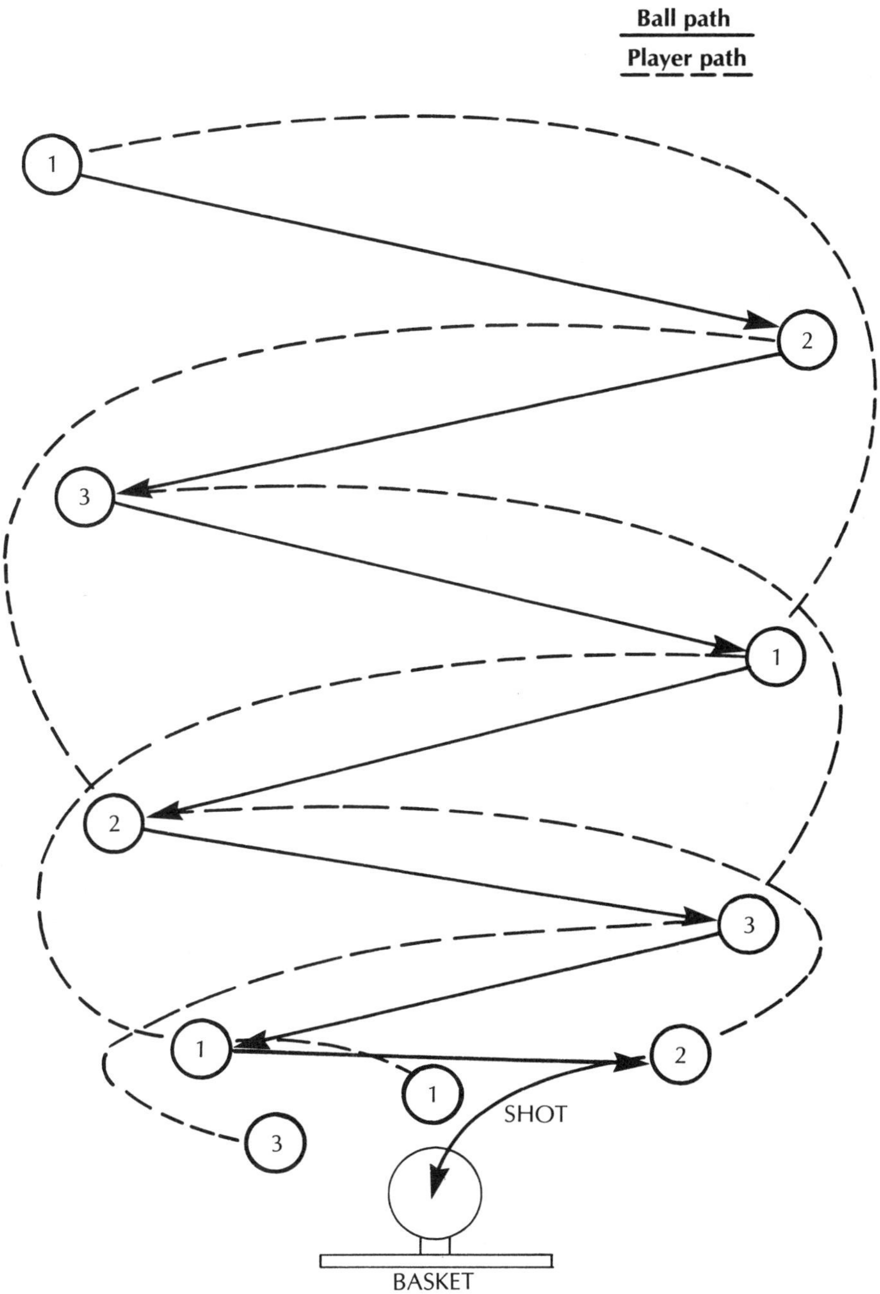

Decision-making is changing input to output

DECISION-MAKING is the label applied to the operation of transforming or changing information taken from the environment (INPUT) into an appropriate movement response (OUTPUT). Like INPUT, DECISION-MAKING involves a number of individual sub-operations which improve with practice. We need to be concerned with:

- interpreting the output;
- deciding on a particular response;
- coordinating the response.

Output is the actual execution of a movement

OUTPUT is the label applied to the actual execution of the movement. It is the execution of the motor response that has been chosen (DECISION-MAKING) as the best or most appropriate in the present situation. Most of the preparation for the output has already been accomplished by the time the movement is in progress but adjustments may be made as performance occurs if this is necessary. (A baseball batter, for example, can stop the swing in midstream if the pitch is judged to be a ball rather than a strike. The decision to stop is made early enough in the sequence of events from input to output.)

Feedback is information about the output

FEEDBACK is a term applied to the information available during or after the movement. It may be information either about the movement, i.e., how the response was done, or about the effect of the movement on the environment, i.e., what was the outcome? Aspects are:

- types of feedback;
- using feedback to change performance;
- special kinds of feedback.

Summary

In order to improve the accuracy and efficiency of motor performance the player must decide what factors lead to successful performance and then practice in ways which will enhance improvement of those factors. In addition the player must learn to integrate the various factors associated with successful performance, e.g., INPUT, DECISION-MAKING, OUTPUT, and FEEDBACK. This book is designed to provide an understanding of the factors that influence learning and performance. The goal is to provide suggestions for how the learning of motor skills might be approached so that the performance improves and the success rate increases.

CHAPTER TWO

achievement

CLASSIFICATION

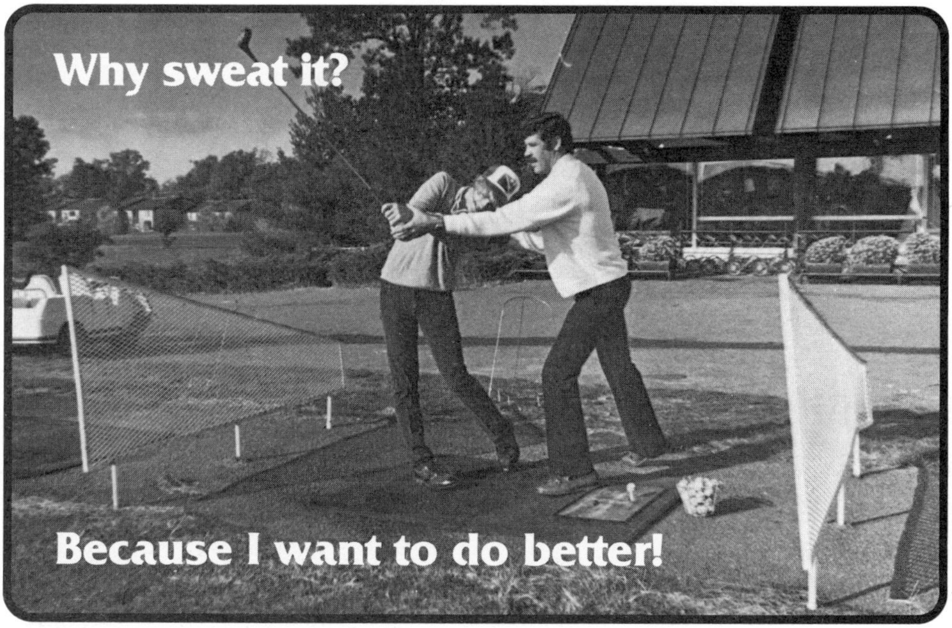

Photograph by Carlyjane Dunn Rice

What Do You Have To Help Me?

Skills come in a variety of types

Skills used in sports and active games come in a variety of types. The differences among the types of skills influence:

- practice procedures;
- focus of attention (concentration);
- decisions about how to respond;
- when to respond;
- what kind of feedback will be most helpful;
- the ease with which a new skill is learned.

Before going on to detail the "types" of skills to be considered, two different types of skills will be reviewed with reference to the items listed above. The skills to be considered are the golf drive and baseball batting.

The type of skill affects practice, attention response, feedback, and cues

Practice. Practice of the golf drive should emphasize *consistency* of ball height, body position in relation to the ball and the flag, club position, body stance, head position, grip, path and speed of backswing, downswing, contact, and follow-through. The golfer attempts to "groove" the swing to establish a consistent, repetitive swing. This is accomplished by intensive practice under constant conditions. This enables a player to develop a consistent swing pattern. Once this consistent swing pattern is established the player uses it with a variety of clubs and a variety of stances and ball positions to accomplish the goal of getting the ball to the green under a variety of circumstances. The swing does not change to meet changing conditions; it remains consistent.

Practicing baseball batting, by contrast, emphasizes development of the player's ability to execute a swing which matches the place and time of the ball's arrival over the plate. In order to enable the batter to develop this skill the practice session must incorporate changes in ball speed and ball flight. Inconsistency in the ball speed and ball flight should be the rule. Practice serves to enable a player to learn to differentiate and interpret the speed and direction of the incoming object and to plan an appropriate response. For this reason a variety of speed and flight combinations should be used. Attention will be given to organizing practice for most effective learning in Chapter Three.

Attention focus. In the golf drive the attention focus should be on the position of the body and the club head with respect to the flag in the address phase and on the rhythm and path of the swing in the action phase. In a word, *inward*, on the totality of the movement. In baseball batting, however, the attention focus should be on the moving ball, *outward*, on the input factors that *must* guide the movement.

Decision-making. There is a difference in how decisions are made as well as in the speed with which they need to be made. In the golf drive the decisions regarding club, stance, club head position, grip, etc., may be made slowly and deliberately. In theory the golfer can take as long as necessary to reach a decision. The particular swing is a consistent, well-used one and is probably not chosen from among a variety of options but rather the golfer accomodates the swing by adjusting the stance and the grip for each particular situation.

In baseball batting, on the other hand, the batter has very little time to decide what is happening and what to do about it.

The distance from the mound to the plate is 90 feet. If a ball travels at 80 mph it takes .77 seconds for the ball to reach the plate once it leaves the pitcher's hand (that is a bit less than 8/10's of a second or less time than it takes to say "swing now"). The process of swinging the bat takes about 4/10's of a second leaving a bit less than 4/10's of a second for the batter to observe the ball flight, decide when and where the ball will arrive, and what to do about it. If a ball is traveling at 100 mph, it takes about 6/10's of a second to reach the plate, leaving 2/10's of a second for input and decision-making. This is in contrast to the almost unlimited time for a skill like golf.

In addition to the difference in the time the batter must also *select* the best response under the circumstances from a greater variety of possibilities in reaching a decision. Clearly the first decision is easy; there are only two choices, swing or don't swing. If the batter decides to swing, the movement selected or structured must meet the time-space constraints imposed by the ball flight and must be chosen from among several alternatives. The task of the batter is weighted more upon decision-making while that of the golfer is weighted more upon the response output.

Response. Following the line of thinking above, it is clear that in golf the performer can respond whenever he or she is ready while in baseball batting the flight of the ball dictates when the response must be initiated and how long it can take.

Feedback. In golf, information about the swing and movement can be useful in facilitating performance. Information concerning the flight of the ball is helpful but is usually used to assess movement errors. For example if a golfer often whiffs or tops the ball the movement error may be: lack of hip and knee flexion; hyperextension of wrists; tension through legs, shoulders, and arms. Consistent hooking of the ball or topping may be due to the club being taken back too far inside on the take-away.

In batting, by contrast, feedback is used to focus on the relationship between the swing and the ball flight. A batter might have a perfect swing but if it is not matched to the ball flight characteristics it won't do much good.

Learning new skills. The skill developed in golf is probably not readily transferable to other skills. That is, knowing how to play golf will probably not help in the learning of other skills (although it might assist in developing the ability to attend to movement information and to analyze errors). The decision-making skills that are developed in baseball batting, however, may facilitate the performance of other skills which involve contacting moving objects: tennis; racqetball; squash; soccer; field hockey.

How?

The information about different types of skills can be used in several ways:

- to vary the level of the skill to be learned from easy to difficult;
- to recognize similarities and differences among skills to be learned;
- to decide what aspects of skill performance to emphasize during practice;
- to determine the prerequisites for success in different skills.

When most people think about classifying skills they think in terms of such categories as:

- individual vs. team sports (archery vs. basketball);
- water sports vs. land sports (swimming vs. soccer);
- gross vs. fine motor skills (softball throw vs. billiards);
- endurance vs. strength activities (marathon vs. weight lifting).

Skills are classified in various ways

The categories listed above have been useful in the past for insuring that physical education programs include a wide variety of types of skills and sports. Very often, however, the best coaching methods for varying skills and sports in the same category might be very different. Swimming, surfing, and water skiing are all water sports but the techniques appropriate to teach each, and the abilities needed to succeed at each, are very different. Some other way or ways of classifying skills is needed if the categories are to have meaning in terms of doing better in sport performance.

Information processing through concepts derived from it has provided a basis for several classification schemes. Several of these schemes will be considered and then integrated into an overall view of the skill types learned in sports:

- *open vs. closed skills* — Classification of skills based upon whether, at the simplest level, the environment is stationary or moving during the skill performance, e.g., foul shot vs. 3-person weave in basketball.
- *self-paced vs. externally-paced skills* — Classification of skills based upon whether control of the initiation and timing of movement is within the performer or in the environment, e.g., golf swing vs. baseball batting.

- *body stability vs. body transport* — Classification of skills based upon whether the total body is stationary or moving during the skill execution, e.g., tennis serve vs. lay-up shot.
- *no manipulation vs. manipulation* — Classification of skills based upon whether the individual has to control an implement (tennis racket) or object (basketball) in addition to the total body motion, e.g., running down court in basketball vs. running and dribbling a basketball.
- *complexity of information processing* — Classification of skills on the basis of factors that may vary from simple to complex at each phase of information processing, e.g., playing basketball one-on-one vs. playing basketball three-on-three.

Skills are open if the environment is moving and closed if not

Open vs. Closed skills. Skills may be classified according to the nature of the environment in which they occur with particular reference to how that particular environment controls movement. At one extreme the environment is stationary as in hitting a ball off a batting tee. At the other extreme the environment is moving as in hitting a pitched ball. In the stationary ball instance movement is controlled only by spatial factors such as the height of the ball. In the second instance the movement is controlled by both the height of the ball and the time of arrival. In the first case the performer must swing the bat so that it passes the point in space where the ball is located. When the swing is initiated the speed of the swing is not critical if the height of the swing is matched to the height of the ball on the batting tee.

In the second instance the swing is controlled by the height and speed of the ball. The timing and placement of the swing must match the time of arrival of the ball as well as the height of the ball. The height of the swing must conform to the height of the ball as in the first example but the crucial difference is that the time of initiation of the swing and the speed of the swing is dictated by the ball's speed.

What are some examples of *closed* skills?

In sport there are many examples of closed skills: the football place kicker has to match the kick to the position of the stationary ball; the archer has to match the flight of the arrow to the position and distance of the center of the target; the diver has to match the dive to the distance to the water and the depth of the pool. Skills like these, and others in which the performer's movements must match or conform to spatial factors only are termed *closed skills*. The environment is stationary, fixed, stable. The position of the elements in the environment is the same before and during the skill performance.

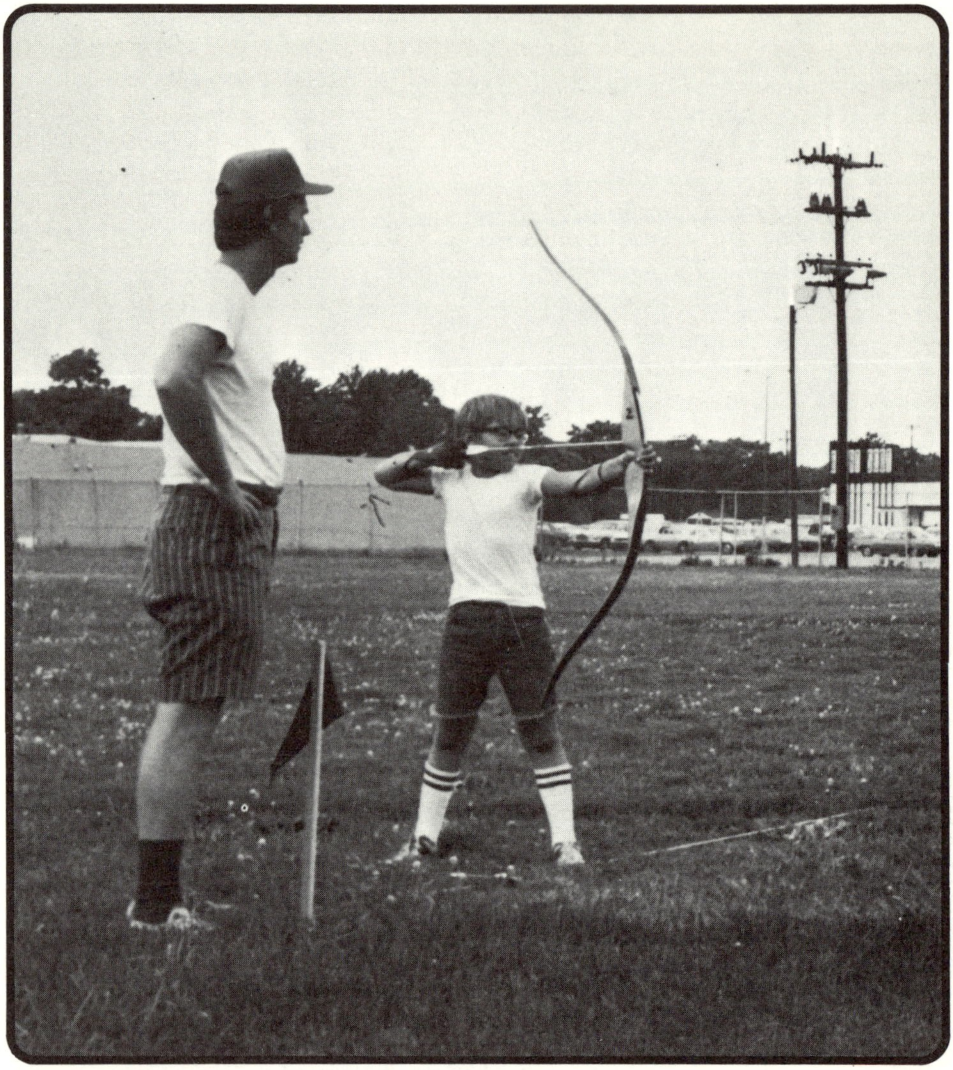

Courtesy of Vigo County School Corporation

Matching the flight of an arrow, in archery, to the position and distance of the center of the target, is an example of a closed skill. The environment is stationary, fixed, stable.

What are some examples of *open* skills?

There are also many examples of open skills. The tennis player has to match the position of the racket and the timing of the forehand drive to the position and speed of the ball; the ice hockey player has to match the position and speed of movement to the position and speed of other players on the team, or that of the opponents, or that of the hockey puck. The basketball player who is dribbling the ball toward the basket must match the path of movement to the position and movement of other players in addition to controlling and matching the movements of the ball. These skills and others like them which demand that movements match the speed, timing, and space of other people or objects are termed *open skills*. The environment in open skills is continually in motion, unstable, and unpredictable.

Environments that are termed *closed* are characterized by the following:

- the spatial elements that control movement do not vary from trial to trial;
- the environment in which performance takes place does not change between the time the skill is planned and the time it is initiated;
- the environment in which performance takes place does not change much from one instance to another;
- movements should be practiced until they become habitual;
- the practice environment should be kept as consistent as possible (at the same time keeping it as much like the. performance environment as possible).

Skills, other than those mentioned previously, which occur in closed environments are archery, bowling, basketball free throw, golf, diving, and gymnastics. What are the spatial elements which control movement in some or all of the skills mentioned? In the case of bowling you might have listed:

- length of the approach;
- width of the approach area;
- distance from the starting position to the foul line;
- position of the pins.

In contrast, environments that are termed *open* are characterized by:

- the time and space elements change from trial to trial and within the trial as when the pitcher throws a change-up;
- the dynamic nature of the environment forces the performer to make predictions about the future time/space features of the environment, e.g., when the pitcher throws the ball, its arrival at the plate must be predicted so that the

swing can be initiated before the ball passes over the plate. See the section on "How can I have good timing?";

- prediction of what will occur each time is based on that which has occurred in the past. If for example a tennis player hits 8 out of 10 shots to the forehand then if the receiver predicts forehand on the next shot he has an 8 out of 10 chance of being correct about the prediction;
- a variety of gamelike situations should be employed so that players can practice *predicting* various heights, speeds, and directions and practice *responding* to those variants.

Open skill environments are controlled by space and time

Suppose you were planning to catch a ball thrown to you. Success in catching a ball requires predicting, during the flight of the ball, where it will arrive and when it will arrive. The hands must then be moved to the predicted place of the ball's arrival. Then at the appropriate instant the closing of the hands must be initiated so that the ball will be trapped. If the hands are closed too early the ball will bounce off the fist. If the hands are closed too late the ball will rebound off the palm of the hand. The timing of the catching response (the grasping phase) must be matched to the arrival time of the ball just as the position of the hand(s) in space must conform to the arrival location of the ball. Thus in open skill environments movements are controlled by the spatial (place) and temporal (time) aspects of the ball's flight. Catching a ball is an open skill because it takes place in an open environment. Other open skills are hitting a baseball, tennis, badminton, playing in a basketball game, soccer game, ice hockey, and field hockey.

Open skill practice requires a varied environment

When open skills are practiced it is best that the situation be varied so that the player learns to respond to a number of different possibilities rather than hitting, for example, a ball tossed to the same location at the same speed and height until the tennis stroke or swing is grooved. Practicing by hitting a consistently tossed ball will almost guarantee that game performance will be poor because:

- the player won't be prepared to discriminate among various ball speeds, heights, and directions;
- the player won't be able to predict the arrival time and place of the ball;
- the player won't be able to plan and initiate a response that fits the situation.

The skills necessary to do those things listed will not have been practiced.

Closed skill practice requires an unvarying environment

For closed skills fine tuning or adjusting the response to an unvarying situation is very appropriate and is in fact desirable. Some closed skills like golf and bowling require a number of

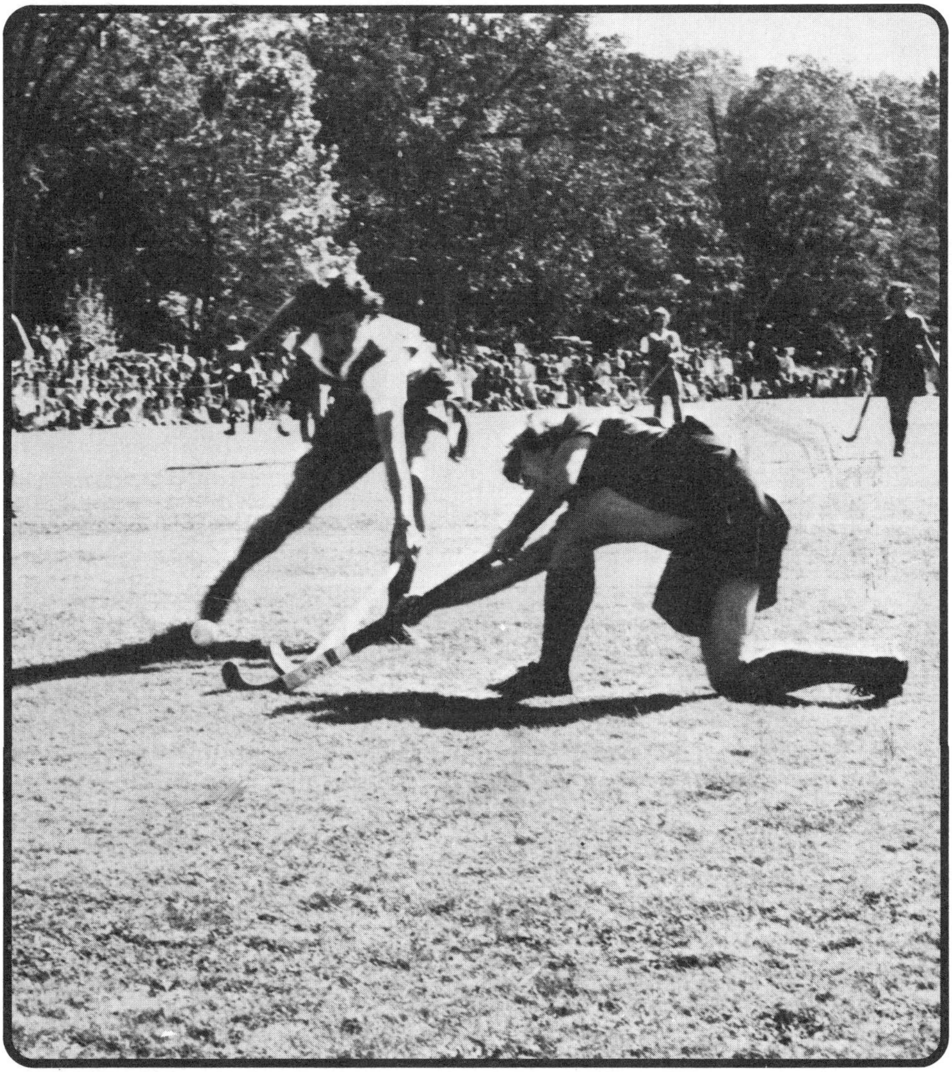

Playing in a field hockey game is an example of an open skill.

different responses to fit some special situations; when the situations occur they are consistent. Even though the setting may change somewhat from trial to trial, each trial nevertheless occurs in a closed environment.

Skills are self-paced if controlled by the performer and externally paced if not

Self-paced vs. Externally-paced. Another way of thinking about skills is in terms of the timing or pacing of the movement. In one instance the timing of the movement initiation and execution is under the performer's control. That is the performer decides when to start the movement and how fast to perform it. These types of movements are termed *self-paced*. For example in the game High Water, Low Water, the rope is stationary and set at a specific height and you decide how fast to approach the rope and how quickly to jump over it. In jumping over a rope that two individuals are turning, however, the speed of the jumping movements and the timing of the jumps themselves is controlled by the speed and height at which the rope is moving. When the rope is quicker, movement must be quicker.

What are self-paced skills? externally-paced skills?

The jump rope example is an externally-paced skill; the rate of movement is *controlled* by the speed of the moving rope. In externally-paced movements, in contrast to self-paced movements, the performer needs to attend more closely to the external events (the rope, the other players, the ball) so that the pace of movement will match the pace of the external events. In externally-paced skills, as in open skills, what the movement looks like is not critical as long as it is efficient, matches the controls imposed by the environment, and accomplishes the goal.

The major difference between open skills and those termed externally-paced is that the former category includes both spatial and temporal aspects while the latter refers to the timing of the movements. The same is true of self-paced and closed. The former includes only time aspects while the latter includes both time and space.

Body stability skills are performed in a stationary position and body transport skills in a moving position

Body Stability vs. Body Transport. In our discussion of open vs. closed and self-paced vs. externally-paced skills we did not specify what the learner was doing (standing still or moving, for example). A skill performed in a stationary position (body stability) is simpler than a similar skill performed when moving (body transport). In a stationary position there is one less element to consider in movement planning and one less element to demand attention. Bouncing a basketball while standing still is easier than running and dribbling at the same time. In the first instance only the movement of the ball demands attention. In the second instance two elements demand attention, movement of the ball and the movement of the body with respect to the ball. The movement of the ball must be coordinated with the running movements or vice versa. In general, adding total body movement to a skill performance makes that performance more complex.

A skill can be simplified during the learning process by attempting it *briefly* while standing in a stationary position. Once the idea is clear try it while moving. In learning to pass in basketball the learner might attempt the following steps:

Movement makes the task of performing a skill more difficult

- stand still and try the pass to a stationary receiver;
- run and pass to a stationary receiver;
- dribble and pass to a stationary receiver;
- dribble and pass to a moving receiver;
- dribble and pass to a moving receiver while being guarded;
- dribble and pass to a moving receiver who is being guarded, while being guarded.

It is most important that the learner doesn't spend too much time on each of these steps but that each is done long enough to get the idea of what is required. The most important practice is that undertaken in game or gamelike situations. Adding movement makes the task of performing a skill more difficult.

Some skills require manipulation of objects

No-Manipulation vs. Manipulation. Another aspect that adds to the complexity of skills that has not been specifically considered in previous discussion concerns manipulation of implements, balls, with the hands, feet, or head. In sports like archery and golf which are closed skills or implements, the bow and arrow and the golf club respectively must be controlled by the arms and hands to accomplish the task. In field hockey and tennis, which are open skills, the hockey stick and the tennis racquet respectively must be manipulated to accomplish the task. This is different from track, a closed skill, in which there is no need to manipulate objects, or basketball, an open skill, in which only one player has control of the ball at a time. A skill which does not involve manipulating or controlling an object or an implement is one less to think about, one less element to control, one less aspect to demand attention.

It is sometimes helpful to think of the manipulation of implements or objects as a *secondary task*. That is one which is done in addition to the principle or primary task of body stability or body transport. Stability and transport are considered to be primary tasks because they provide the base of

Manipulation of objects involves the primary task of body stability or transport and the secondary task involving manipulation

support from which all the aspects of manipulation occur. If the primary task is not performed well, then adding another task will cause performance in the primary task to worsen. As an illustration suppose an individual was asked to run through a complicated obstacle course and the time it took to complete the course was used as the measure of performance. If the same individual was then asked to run through the course while dribbling a basketball the time to complete the course would increase. The addition of the secondary task, dribbling the basketball, increased the time necessary to do the primary task, running the obstacle course. The primary task demanded a certain attention level; when the secondary task was added attention was diverted and shared between the primary and the secondary task thus affecting the performance of the total task.

As skill in the primary task increases, it demands less attention. At later stages of learning the performance of the primary task (transport or stability) becomes semi-automatic and attention can be diverted to the secondary task without a noticeable affect on overall performance.

Complexity of a skill may influence any or all of the information processing aspects

Complexity of Information Processing. A final consideration in classification of skills relates to the four information processing operations mentioned previously: INPUT, DECISION-MAKING, OUTPUT, and FEEDBACK. The complexity of the INPUT phase can vary depending upon the number of critical stimuli, the speed of events, and other factors listed in Table 2.1. In similar fashion the complexity of the DECISION-MAKING phase can vary. Likewise, the OUTPUT and FEEDBACK phases can differ.

Most of the complexity can be controlled in practice, but in the game the factors will have certain values. In basketball for example:

- there are many critical stimuli;
- there is a high ratio between critical and non-critical stimuli;
- events occur at fast speed;
- there are many confusing stimuli;
- many factors must be considered in planning the response;
- there are many alternative choices and the distinctions among them are subtle;
- the times between input/decision-making and decision-making/execution are short;
- the movements require the coordination of many body parts simultaneously.

Table 2.1: Analyzing Complexity of Information Processing

Minimum	COMPLEXITY	Maximum
	INPUT	
FEW	Number of critical stimuli	MANY
LOW (1:1)	Ratio between critical: non-critical stimuli	HIGH (1:10)
SLOW	The speed at which events occur	FAST
HIGH	The intensity of the stimuli	LOW
HIGH	Contrast between critical and non-critical stimuli	LOW
FEW	Amount of confusing stimuli	MANY
LONG	Length of break between individual events	SHORT
	DECISION-MAKING	
FEW	Number of factors to be considered	MANY
FEW	Number of alternative choices	MANY
SMALL	Amount of information needed	LARGE
LONG	Time between input/decision-making and decision-making/output	SHORT
	OUTPUT	
FEW	Number of sequential or simultaneous movements	MANY
FEW	Number of body parts involved	MANY
LOW	Precision required	HIGH
LARGE	Size of base of support	SMALL
SIMPLE	Rhythmic structure of movement	COMPLEX
	FEEDBACK	
SMALL	Amount of information available	LARGE
FEW	Number of transformations before using feedback	MANY
AVERAGE	Precision of information	LOW or HIGH

Task difficulty can be reduced by manipulating the task components

The game of tennis by contrast tends toward less complexity:

- there are few critical stimuli;
- the ratio between critical and non-critical stimuli is low;
- the intensity is medium;
- the contrast is medium;
- there are few confusing stimuli;
- there are player-controlled breaks in the action;
- the number of alternative choices is comparatively low.

These complexity factors may be thought of in terms of task difficulty. The difficulty of a task can be reduced by manipulating those aspects related to INPUT, DECISION-MAKING, OUTPUT, and FEEDBACK operations that affect complexity. By categorizing skills according to difficulty those skills which are less complex can be practiced first and then gradually more complex skills can be added. In addition, skills which are complex in some ways but easier in other ways might provide good practice. Finally, a particular skill can be varied in complexity by manipulating appropriate aspects.

Sport Skills – An Integration

Skills performed in sport situations involve all aspects which have been discussed:

- the environment may be open or closed;
- the performer may need to focus on moving through space or on maintaining a stable position;
- the performer may manipulate an object or implement or perform some other secondary task;
- the complexity of the information processing operations may vary from minimal to maximal.

The level of skill difficulty may be determined in part by analyzing it with respect to the aspects listed.

Complex skills are easier to learn if reduced to a simpler form and then gradually made more complex

The simplest skill may involve a closed environment with no locomotion, no object manipulation, and minimal information processing complexity. The most difficult skill may involve an open environment with locomotion, object manipulation, and maximal information processing complexity. The first example can be illustrated by standing in place in an empty room; the second can be illustrated by dribbling a basketball toward the basket through a group of moving opponents. When learning a skill it may be wise to adjust the skill to a simpler form by eliminating some of the aspects that make it more difficult and then gradually including them as the performer's proficiency increases. In the basketball example above it might be easier to teach a player to dribble without anyone on the court to impede progress or distract attention. Then to encourage the player to watch where he is going, the player should dribble around a set of stationary cones. Finally the player should dribble around players who are permitted to move within limited space. The ultimate test is to use the skill in a game situation.

Summary

Different skills make different demands on "attention" capabilities. Sport skills can be classified according to:

- the environment in which they take place (open or closed);
- the state of your body (stationary or moving);
- the presence of a secondary task (manipulation or no-manipulation);
- the complexity of information processing (minimal or maximal);

Some skills allow total concentration on movement. Other skills require concentration on both movement and the moving environment. In still others the player must move through a moving environment possibly avoiding other moving people while swinging a tennis racket, dribbling a soccer ball, or performing some other attention demanding task. Some of the most difficult sport skills are in the last category; some of the simplest are in the first. There are, however, skills of varying degrees of difficulty in all of the categories; these may be assessed by evaluation of complexity. A one-handed handstand is in the same environment, body and manipulation category as standing in place although the handstand is clearly more difficult. The base of support is smaller making the output more complex.

In modifying movements or skills to make them easier to perform it should be remembered that although it is possible to practice open skills in closed environments, for example, *extensive* practice of this type is not likely to be very effective. Therefore this type of modification should be used minimally if at all and then only with specific goals in mind.

Are closed skills really easier?

Finally, although closed skills may be the easiest skills to perform when environmental complexity is considered some closed skills demand extraordinary qualities of movement sense (kinesthesis) and movement control on the part of the performer. Therefore the skills of gymnasts, divers, figure

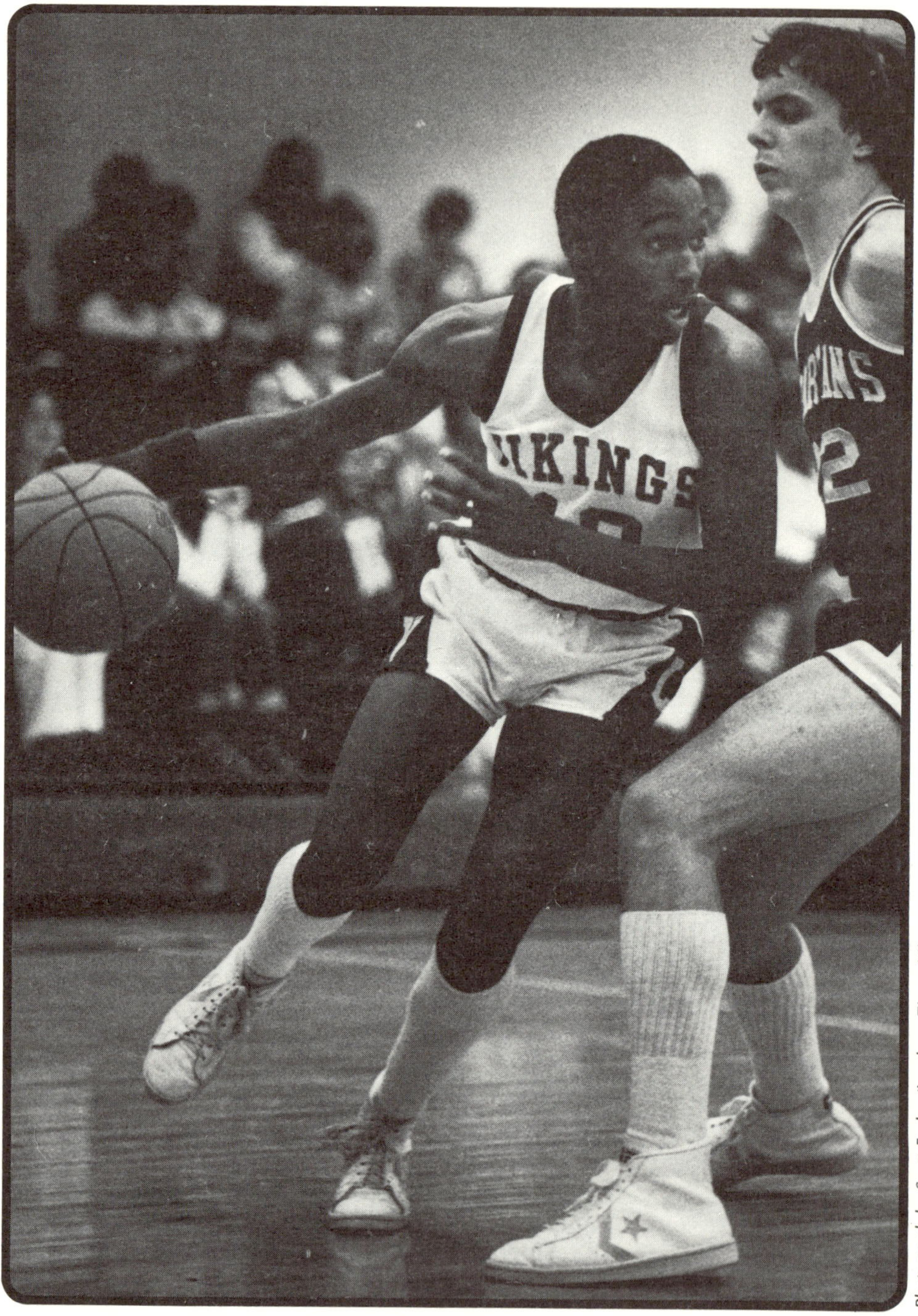

Photograph by Scott Forbes/Loudoun Times-Mirror

In basketball, dribbling around players who are permitted to move within limited space involves an open environment with locomotion, object manipulation, and maximal information processing complexity.

skaters, and the like should not be underestimated because the environment is stationary and because different abilities than those required in open skills are critical to success. Rather each successful participant should be regarded with awe because he or she has been able to put it all together in optimal fashion.

CHAPTER THREE

achievement

PRACTICE

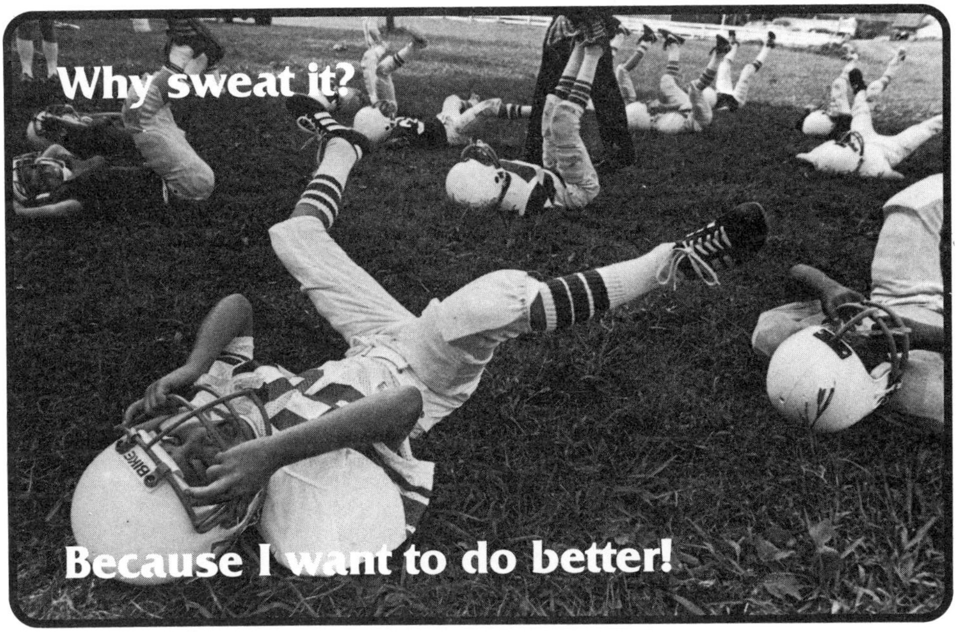

Photograph by Scott Forbes/Loudoun Times-Mirror

What Do You Have To Help Me?

One means of doing better is to PRACTICE. Although the notion that "practice makes perfect" is not quite true (feedback is necessary for improvement in skill performance) it is clear that:

NO PRACTICE = NO IMPROVEMENT.

The question that must be answered, however, is "How should practice be organized for the greatest improvement to occur?"

How **the learner practices is the key to improving performance**

Since practice is an investment of time and effort, individuals should be concerned with getting the best possible return on their investment. There are several alternative methods for practicing. In some instances one method of practice is clearly better than its opposing method but this is not typical. Rather the superiority of one method over another may depend on:

- the type of skill to be learned;
- the amount of time alloted for practice;
- the goal of the activity;
- the characteristics of the individual learning the skill.

In spite of these qualifications it is useful and important to be aware of the practice options available. Each of the options to be considered is presented below and briefly defined. Then each option is discussed in more detail with respect to the choices within that option and the differences among the possible choices in terms of return on the practice investment.

Should the goal of practice be to perform as quickly as possible or to perform as accurately as possible?
Skills which involve both speed of movement and accuracy of outcome may be practiced in ways which emphasize either or both of these characteristics. For example in pitching a baseball the pitcher may be told to throw for the strike (emphasize accuracy) or to throw for speed (emphasize movement speed) or to throw as quickly and accurately as possible.

Should skills be practiced in their entirety or in segments?
Skills may be viewed as consisting of a number of segments or parts. In practicing new skills these parts may be practiced separately or as a whole unit. In executing a lay-up shot in basketball, for example, the learner may practice the shot, the take-off, the approach, and the dribble separately or as a single unit. Practicing in parts is called "part" practice, while practicing in one unit is called "whole" practice.

Should practice be continuous (without resting) or should it be in short, frequent units?
The time allotted to practice a skill may be used in one continuous block or it may be divided into a number of smaller segments. Practicing a skill in one continuous block of time or in several large blocks is called "massed" practice. Practicing the skill in a number of smaller segments with rest periods between practices is called "distributed" practice. In using a total practice time of 2 hours per week a coach may have the team practice for 2 hours on a single day or for one half hour on each of 4 days. The latter schedule would be called distributed, the former massed.

Should practice involve actually doing the skill or can it involve imagining doing the skill?
Skills are usually practiced by actually doing them but it is possible to improve by imagining undertaking the skill. The actual practice is called physical practice, while imaginal practice is called mental practice. The golf drive might be

learned by going to the driving range and actually hitting 200 balls per day, or by spending one day imagining hitting 200 golf balls.

How?

Practice for speed, for accuracy, or for both as the skill requires

Speed versus accuracy. There are three choices in relation to the *speed and accuracy* of skill performance. The skill can be performed:

- as quickly as possible as in pitching a fast ball;
- as accurately as possible as in pitching the ball into the strike zone every time;
- as quickly *and* accurately as possible as in pitching the ball fast *and* into the strike zone;

Usually individuals refer to a speed-accuracy trade-off. This means that in order to be as accurate as possible the skill must be performed more slowly. To perform as fast as possible accuracy will have to be sacrificed. When both speed and accuracy are emphasized then both are attained to a more moderate degree.

For some time individuals believed that the best way to learn a skill was to practice it slowly at first, emphasizing the accuracy of the movement and then gradually increasing the speed until it reached an acceptable level. It was believed that at slower speeds the performer could be very accurate in the movement because the progress of the movement could be controlled. It was suggested that the performer could monitor the progress of the movement throughout and make adjustments as necessary.

The application of this suggestion to a sport skill, bowling for instance, would dictate that the beginning bowler should move slowly and deliberately during the approach and delivery so that movements could be monitored and adjustments made as required. An alternative would be for the bowler to attempt to adjust the delivery so that the ball travels down the alley as fast as possible. Neither of these methods would be wholly satisfactory.

The best way to practice the skill of bowling would be to use a moderate speed of delivery and also attempt to maintain a moderate degree of accuracy. A performer will need to explore combinations of speed and accuracy until the right combination for him and the skill is attained. While bowling may demand more accuracy and less speed, pitching a baseball may demand more speed and less accuracy. In spite of the fact that most tennis coaches indicate that the second serve should be as fast as the first, most intermediate players and some advanced players will cut down on the speed of the second serve to insure accuracy.

The size of the target generally has an effect on the speed-accuracy trade-off. To test or demonstrate this notion several individuals might participate in a brief game. Make or draw several targets of different sizes and give each person ten chances at each target emphasizing that the balls should be thrown with both speed and accuracy. Do they throw at the same speed for all targets? If they do are they more accurate at some than at others? If they do not do they tend to throw more slowly at the smaller targets or at the bigger targets?

Figure 3.1 illustrates the notion of the speed-accuracy trade-off. Skills which demand high accuracy but not high speed are to the left; skills which demand high speed but not high accuracy are at the right; skills which demand both are toward the center. In bowling, pitching, and tennis the best results would be obtained when both speed and accuracy are moderate; for throwing events in track and field, speed of movement is more critical than accuracy so speed would be emphasized as it would in the tennis or badminton smash. In the drop shot or hairpin shot in badminton, however, placement accuracy is foremost and so this would be emphasized at the expense of speed. What are other skills or sports in which accuracy is emphasized at the expense of speed?, speed at the expense of accuracy?, speed and accuracy equally?

In summary emphasis on speed and/or accuracy requires a trade-off. Individuals cannot perform at top speed and be optimally accurate also. Speed must be reduced to gain accuracy, and accuracy is lost when speed is gained. Each performer in consultation with his teacher or coach must decide what is important in the performance of the particular activity to be learned or practiced and then attention must be focused on speed, accuracy, or both as appropriate to optimal success.

What Else?

A skill may be practiced in its entirety or it may be broken down into its parts and each part practiced separately. In swimming for example the whole stroke may be practiced as a single unit or it may be practiced in parts (arms, legs, breathing) and then combined into the total stroke. The lay-up shot

Figure 3.1: An Illustration of the Speed-Accuracy Trade-Off.

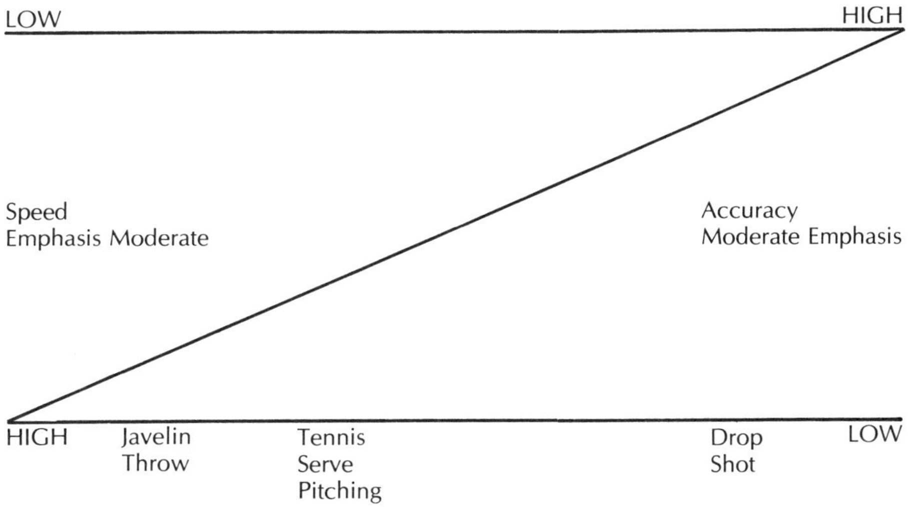

may be practiced as a single unit or it may be practiced in parts (the dribble, the approach, the take-off, the shot) and then combined into the total skill. Finally volleyball students may be put into a game situation and expected to learn all the different skills of the game through playing the whole game or each of the individual skills, the set, the serve, the pass, the spike, and the block, may be taught and drilled individually before the learner is allowed to play the game.

Three situations were used to illustrate the point because the three situations are slightly different and these differences have a bearing on the way they should be practiced. The swimming stroke is an example of a skill in which the parts occur simultaneously; in the lay-up the parts occur in sequence; in volleyball the game is composed of a number of independent skills.

In swimming, the arm action, the leg action, and the breathing action are rhythmically related. In the crawl there are three leg actions for each arm action, and one breath to each two arm actions. In skills like swimming in which the parts are rhythmically related, practice contributes to learning the individual parts and the rhythmical relationship among the parts. What are some other skills in which the parts occur simultaneously? Fencing, dance, and bowling are good examples.

In the lay-up shot in basketball the actions take place in some predetermined sequence. All the parts of the skill are related in that the segments have a particular relationship in sequence and in timing; successful execution requires that this relationship be maintained. In skills such as the lay-up shot the performer not only learns the parts of the skill and their sequence but also the intersegment timing. What are other skills in which the segments take place in a particular sequence and the intersegment timing is critical? The tennis serve, the foul shot, the archery draw and release would be good examples.

Finally the skills in the *game* of volleyball bear little relationship to one another and so may be considered as independent skills. Each skill is distinct from the others and in fact may be either a sequential or simultaneous skill. However they are related because together they constitute the game of volleyball. These skills must be learned as individual skills but they must also be learned in relationship to each other and to the total game of volleyball. Each particular skill is specifically related to the total game in some way. What are some other games in which the skills are independent? Basketball, tennis, or badminton are games comprised of independent skills.

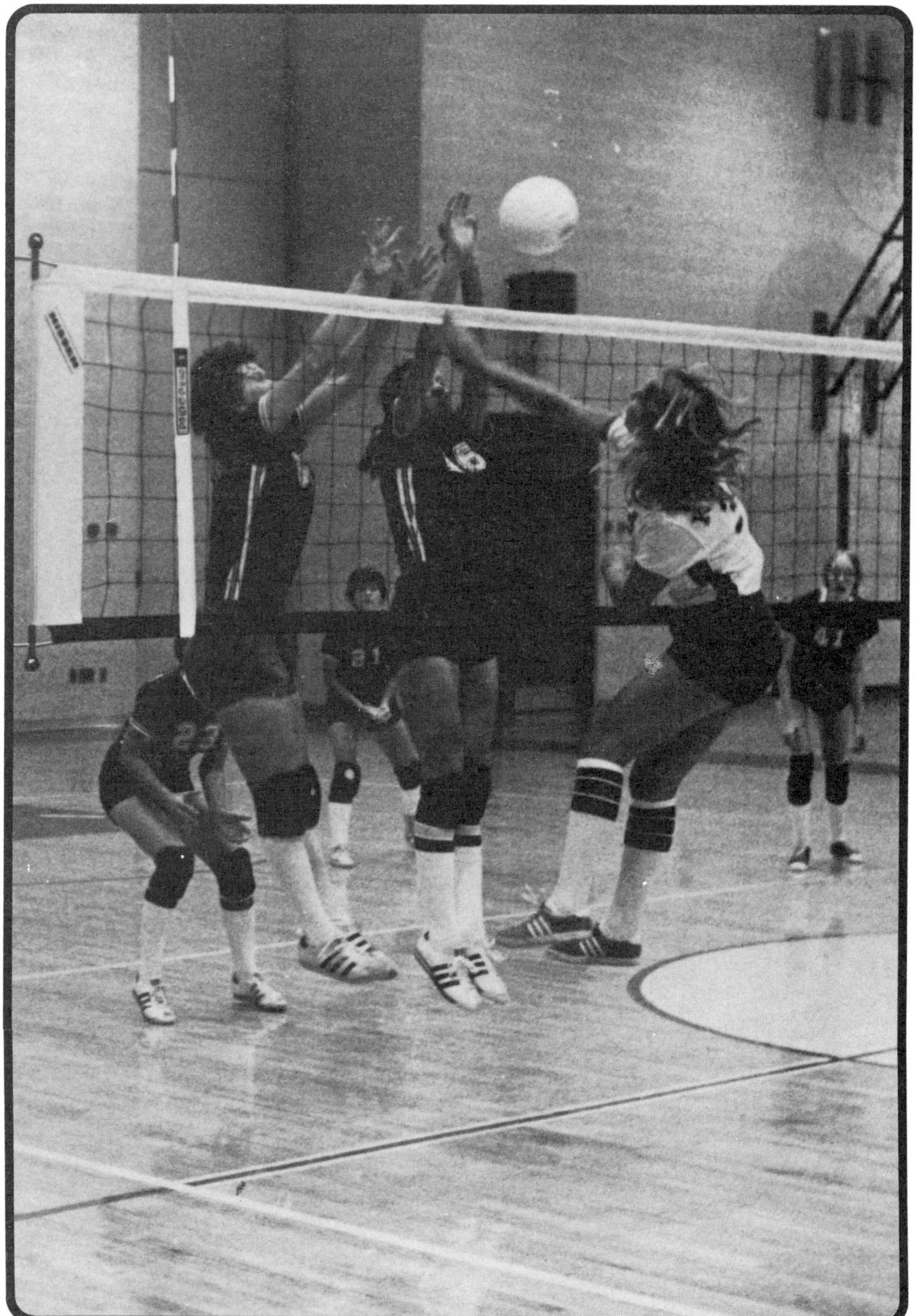

Each skill, in a game of volleyball is distinct from the others and may be considered independent skills.

Skills in which the parts are simultaneous are usually best practiced by the whole method

Skills in which the parts of the skill are simultaneous are usually best learned and practiced by the whole method. That is wherever possible the skill should be performed in total as a single unit. When necessary a portion of the skill, e.g., the leg action in swimming, may be isolated and practiced briefly but it should immediately be incorporated back into the complete stroke. As was mentioned previously the integration and rhythmic coordination of the parts contributes to successful performance in simultaneous skills. It is this aspect that is practiced during the whole practice. While the teacher may wish to have a student exercise a particular element in isolation, extensive practice in refining an aspect of a simultaneous skill without emphasis on the integration of the refined part into the whole may be detrimental to performance of the total skill.

Which skills require whole practice? part practice?

In the case of a sequential skill where the parts follow in a particular order (as in folk dance, a gymnastics routine, or the lay-up in basketball), the skill should be analyzed to ascertain whether the parts can be easily identified and whether they are meaningful and distinct in isolation. In the case of folk dances and gymnastics routines the parts are often meaningful (they can stand alone as independent skills). In the case of the lay-up shot it is less likely that the parts as suggested previously, are meaningful apart from the rest. When the parts of the skill are not distinct and cannot stand alone it is best to practice the whole skill as a total unit with allowance for extra brief attention to a particular aspect if needed.

Skills should be practiced in part if a skill is intricate and/or long and/or the learner is very young

Another consideration in the case of a sequential skill is the length of the total skill. This may also be related to the memory and attention capacity of the learner. If the total folk dance, for example, is short and the students have the capacity to retain all of the steps then it is probably best to practice the total dance. If the dance is long, the parts intricate, or the memory and attention capacity of the learners warrant, then the skill should be presented and practiced in parts.

Often in sequential skills a technique known as progressive part is used to present and practice the skill. In a folk dance with five distinct and independent segments the teacher presents step one and the learners practice step one. Then step two is presented and the learners practice steps one and two. Step three is presented and the learners practice one, two, and three. This method of practice continues until all of the parts have been learned. One problem with this technique of course is that the initial portions of the skill, having been reviewed and practiced the most often, are best learned. An

Whole-part-whole practice is best for sports comprised of many independent skills

advantage to learning this way rather than by the strict part method is that the learner learns the parts as well as the transitions from one part to the next.

In the case of a sport comprised of independent skills (volleyball, tennis, and badminton, among others) it is best to use what is termed the whole-part-whole technique possibly in a mini-game or controlled game situation. For example the spike in volleyball is first presented in a game situation in which students are given the opportunity to briefly attempt the skill. Then with the knowledge of its relationship to the game the students are prepared to learn and practice the skill in a short drill situation before continuing practice in a mini-game or controlled game or game-like drill. Finally the students will incorporate the skill into the game possibly with the stipulation that only points resulting from a successful spike will count, thus encouraging the use of that skill. See Table 3.1 for a summary of factors influencing whole-part.

What Else?

Massed vs. distributed practice

Another aspect of concern is the amount of time the skill is practiced as it relates to the number and placement of the rest periods. Sometimes in class, for example, the number of attempts at a skill or the amount of time at a particular task is dictated by the teacher and by the number of students sharing the equipment and facilities. At other times during class or after school on the playground the performer can establish an individual time schedule. She can choose to spend a long time practicing, taking many attempts, or she can take a few attempts and spend a short time practicing. A performer might also choose to spend a long time practicing but might take frequent breaks during that time for practice, rest, practice, rest, and so on.

Practice time should vary according to difficulty and type of skill and age of the learner

Suppose a coach wishes to schedule team practices, any sport will serve as an example: basketball, golf, volleyball, track, gymnastics. Practice could be set up any number of ways. The team members might practice two hours a day, twice a week, and during those two hours might work or play constantly, scrimmaging or performing for the total two hours with only game-related pauses. Alternatively the team members might practice only 50 minutes per day but practice every day. The time spent in practice is almost the same, 240 minutes in the first instance as compared with 250 minutes in

Table 3.1: Factors which influence choice of whole or part practice.

Practice should/can emphasize:

	Wholes	*Parts*
If the task:	*Has highly dependent (integrated) parts.*	*Has highly independent parts.*
	Is simple.	*Is made up of individual skills.*
	Is not meaningful in parts.	*Is very complex.*
	Is made up of simultaneously performed parts.	*If limited work on parts or different segments is necessary.*
If the learner:	*Is able to remember long sequences.*	*Has a limited memory span.*
	Has a long attention span.	*Is not able to concentrate for a long period of time.*
	Is highly skilled.	*Is having difficulty with a particular part.*
		Cannot succeed with the whole method.

the latter case. The first would be called massed practice because the time blocks are longer; the second would be called distributed because practice is shorter and more frequent. As another alternative, practice might entail 90 minutes a day every day, with a 13 minute workout alternating with 12 minute rests for a total of 260 minutes of practice per week. This would also be distributed practice.

The evidence regarding the time distribution of practice is somewhat difficult to interpret due to:

- the manner in which massed and distributed are defined;
- the age of the students;
- the type of skill to be learned.

Nevertheless certain factors can be helpful in deciding how much time to allot to practicing a particular task and how to organize that time. Some suggested guidelines are presented in Table 3.2. In the case of a gymnastics routine, check the table to find out where gymnastics might fit. In gymnastics optimal, safe performance often involves considerable warm-up of the various muscles of the body. In addition the total routine is usually complex and consists of many elements. Therefore the practice time should be comparatively long since time for warming up and time for practicing the routine must be included. For this reason 1½-2½ hours several times per week may be more appropriate than 1 hour at more frequent intervals. For the basketball foul shot, a repetitive and sometimes boring skill, frequent, shorter, practice periods would be appropriate. This does not necessarily mean that an individual would go to the court each day and spend 10-20 minutes practicing the foul shot. Instead an entire workout in which each of several basketball skills are practiced for a short interval several times during the practice session would be most suitable. An example of how this might be done is shown in Table 3.3. Each skill would be practiced in a realistic, game-like setting. The placement and frequency of each skill might be varied according to the needs of the individual players.

Practicing when over fatigued is a waste of time

Continuing practice when a player is so tired that he can hardly move can be detrimental in terms of the return on the practice investment. This is a major consideration when selecting massed or distributed practice. The length, organization, and frequency of practices should be adjusted to suit the performer and the skill that is to be learned and practiced.

Table 3.2: Factors which may influence your choice of massed or distributed practice organizations.

	Shorter and More Frequent	Longer and Less Frequent
If the task:	is simple, repetitive boring	is complex
	demands intense concentration	has many elements
		requires warm-up
	is fatiguing	is a new one for the performer
	demands close attention to detail	
If the learner:	is young or immature (unable to sustain activity)	is older or more mature
	has a short attention span	is able to concentrate for long periods of time
	has poor concentration skills	has good ability to focus attention
	fatigues easily	tires quickly

Table 3.3: Sample time distribution for a practice.

3:00 p.m.	Practice begins
3:00 p.m.	Warm-up, sprints, stretching, calisthenics, jogging around gym
3:15 p.m.	Sprints with dribbling
3:25 p.m.	Foul shot practice
3:35 p.m.	Lay-up drill
3:45 p.m.	Shots from floor, one-on-one
3:50 p.m.	Full scrimmage
4:10 p.m.	Foul shot practice
4:20 p.m.	Chalk talk, new plays, problems, questions
4:40 p.m.	Floor shots one-on-one
4:45 p.m.	Full scrimmage
5:05 p.m.	Sprints
5:10 p.m.	Foul shots
5:15 p.m.	Cool-down exercises
5:30 p.m.	Practice ends

What Else?

Mental practice can improve performance

Combining mental and physical practice can result in maximum improvement

Incredible as it may seem it is possible to improve on the performance of a skill by simply imagining or visualizing the performance of that skill. Don't be misled by this claim, however, because it is much better to practice a skill by actually doing it; imagining the performance is better than not practicing at all. It is also true that a combination of doing and imagining can sometimes result in more improvement than just physically practicing. Going through the motions of performing a skill by using the imagination is called *mental practice*. It is important to note that during mental practice there is no observable movement. Actually performing or doing the skill is called *physical practice*.

Mental practice works best for skilled performers with familiar closed skills

Although many individuals have investigated the role that mental practice plays in the learning of a skill the majority of them have tested mental practices using closed or self-paced skills. Mental practice works well with closed skills but not as well as physical practice. A combination of mental practice and physical practice used in an alternating fashion seems to be as good as or better than physical practice alone. If mental practice is used to rehearse open skills then the moving object must also be imagined. Mental practice in combination with equal amounts of physical practice, seems to work with open skills in the few studies where it has been tested.

Mental practice seems to work best if the skill to be performed is familiar. Individuals who are highly skilled seem to have more success with mental practice than those individuals who are novices at the skill. Although it is sometimes helpful to have some direction, possibly in the form of verbal or written cues, it is usually best if cues are used sparingly in combination with non-cued mental practice. Sometimes individuals who use mental practice tally each mental attempt to perform the skill (in mentally shooting foul shots, for example, the student would score one point for each shot that went through the basket). This is motivating and also helps keep track of how many attempts have been taken. Strange as it may seem individuals using mental practice do not always achieve a "perfect" score. In fact the types of scores reported for mental practice trials are very similar to those obtained in actual practice.

In addition to the potential of mental practice for skill acquisition it can be used for pre-performance rehearsal of a skill before executing it in an athletic competition. High jumpers, golfers, archers, gymnasts, pole vaulters, divers, and others use some form of mental rehearsal of the action prior to execution. It has been suggested that Dwight Stone who won a bronze medal in high jumping at the Montreal Olympics, does not begin his approach until he has rehearsed a successful jump even if it necessitates many rehearsals. In fact TV viewers could almost see his eyes and head move as he visualized the approach, the take-off, and the clearing of the bar.

Summary

Different methods for practicing were discussed in this section. There were no easy answers presented because the choice of "best" practice emphasis or method depends on:

- the skill level of the learner;
- the type of skill to be learned;
- the age of the learner;
- the amount of time available.

Each of these alternatives should be considered when a practice session is planned:

- speed vs. accuracy emphasis;
- whole vs. part emphasis;
- massed vs. distributed emphasis;
- mental vs. physical emphasis.

Becoming aware of these alternatives will enable the teacher or the learner to vary the practice sessions. Change or novelty in the practice sessions often enhances learning of skills because it stimulates concentration to the task being performed. These methods and emphases should be used to further stimulate instruction and practice to maintain interest and concentration.

CHAPTER FOUR

achievement

ALTERNATIVES

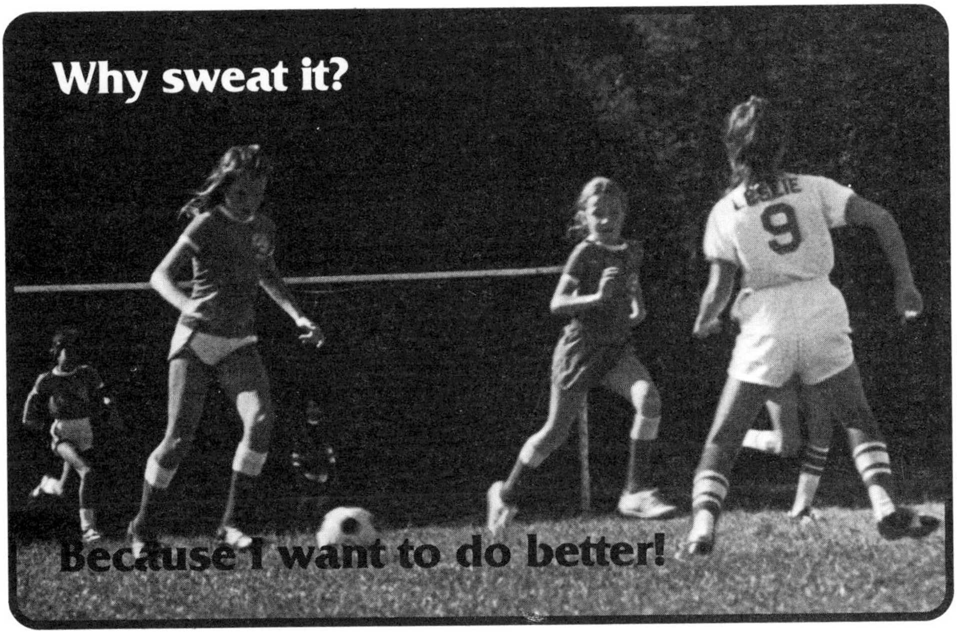

Photograph by Carlyjane Dunn Rice

What Do You Have To Help Me?

Practice methods must be appropriate for the skill to be learned

Practice methods which work for one particular skill are not always equally effective for other skills. Practicing in inappropriate ways for the skill to be learned can *negatively* affect performance (the performer won't learn as much as might have been learned using an appropriate method). Inappropriate practice may lead to poorer performance than no practice. Since more material is available on skills which take place in open environments versus those that take place in closed environments, that aspect will be considered in detail to illustrate the need for structuring practice in ways that are appropriate to the skill to be learned.

How and Why Does It Happen This Way?

What type of practice works best for open skills? for closed skills?

Open and closed skills make different demands on the performer necessitating the development of different capabilities. Practice of open and closed skills must reflect the different demands if the time and effort spent in that practice is to be worthwhile. Closed skills demand consistent, habitual movement. The environment is fixed, stable, and unchanging and the best choice is to attempt to do the same skill in the same manner each time. Some individuals use the term fixation to indicate that a movement habit that will be successful is fixed or set in matching closed environment demands. In contrast, skills performed in an open environment, i.e., open skills, demand rapid discrimination, interpretation, and anticipation of constantly changing events. The movement must be adapted to the situation of the moment. In baseball the pitcher delivers the ball at different heights and speeds and the batter must discriminate the differences, interpret the information in terms of the arrival place and time of the ball, and adjust the level and timing of the swing to match the particular ball characteristics. In basketball the players shoot from different distances on the court and must adjust the angle and force of their shots to conform to the perceived distance. The need to adapt the movement to the situation of the moment has been termed diversification.

The diagram presented in Figure 4.1A illustrates what occurs during learning in a closed environment. The beginning learner makes a wide variety of responses which have varying degrees of success. With continued practice the variety of responses narrows until the individual executes a habitual response consistently and experiences a high rate of success in goal accomplishment at later learning stages. In this closed skill situation the learner must differentiate both the correct response and the environmental cues which are associated with that response. Since the environment is closed there is sufficient time to do both.

Figure 4.1B depicts learning in an open environment. The beginning learner has difficulty discriminating among sets of environmental cues and among the various responses necessary to match those cues. As learning proceeds the individual is able to discriminate among the various sets of environmental conditions and their respective responses and is finally able to match the appropriate response to its environmental cue set. The more advanced open skill performer has a collection of responses to fit a variety of environmental situations.

Figure 4.1: What occurs during learning of open and closed skills.

Figure 4.1.A: Closed Environment

initially variable responses with inconsistent execution	—— LEARNING ——→	habitual consistent response which conforms to the unchanging invariant environment

Figure 4.1.B: Open Environment

initially diverse, undifferentiated responses made in attempting deal with the changing environment	—— LEARNING ——→	specific responses to match specific environmental conditions

*drawings from Higgins; and Spaeth. "Relationship between consistency of movement and environmental condition." *Quest* 17: 61-69.

Under diverse conditions the open skill athlete develops a "rule" which enables him to formulate a wide variety of responses with sufficient practice.

The important consideration in terms of open and closed skills is, of course, how practice is organized to emphasize fixation or diversification. In the next sections fixation and diversification are considered and examples of the types of skills that would benefit from each type of practice and the methods for achieving the required type of practice are provided.

Fixation

Fixation = consistency

Practice with emphasis on fixation, or sameness of environmental cues, is appropriate for closed skills. In actual performance the environment is stationary, stable, and predictable. In addition there is little if any change from one attempt at performance to the next. It is advantageous to keep the environment the same in practice as it will be in competition or the same in the competition as it was in practice.

Think of the Olympic gymnast Nadia Comenici as she prepares to execute a handspring over the vaulting horse. She paces off the distance from the take-off board to her starting position and meticulously places the take-off board a precise distance from the vaulting horse. The height of the vaulting horse is the same used in her practice sessions. She and her coach make certain that the distances and heights are precisely the same as those she will use in the competition and that they are consistent from vault to vault. When she executes the vault she does not have to adapt her movements to differing heights and distances; she executes the vault precisely as she has done in practice. If her movements match those prescribed by the rules she will receive a maximum score of 10. In practice she attempts to fixate or habituate the precise performance characteristics required by the rules. This is a difficult task though Olympic caliber performers make it appear easy. It should be noted that although the rules which govern awarding of points in gymnastics, figure skating, and diving prescribe movement, each performer may still have his own "style" or manner of performance without fear of losing points.

Skills such as gymnastics, figure skating, and diving, in which your form is scored according to a point system are special types of closed skills because the movement and the

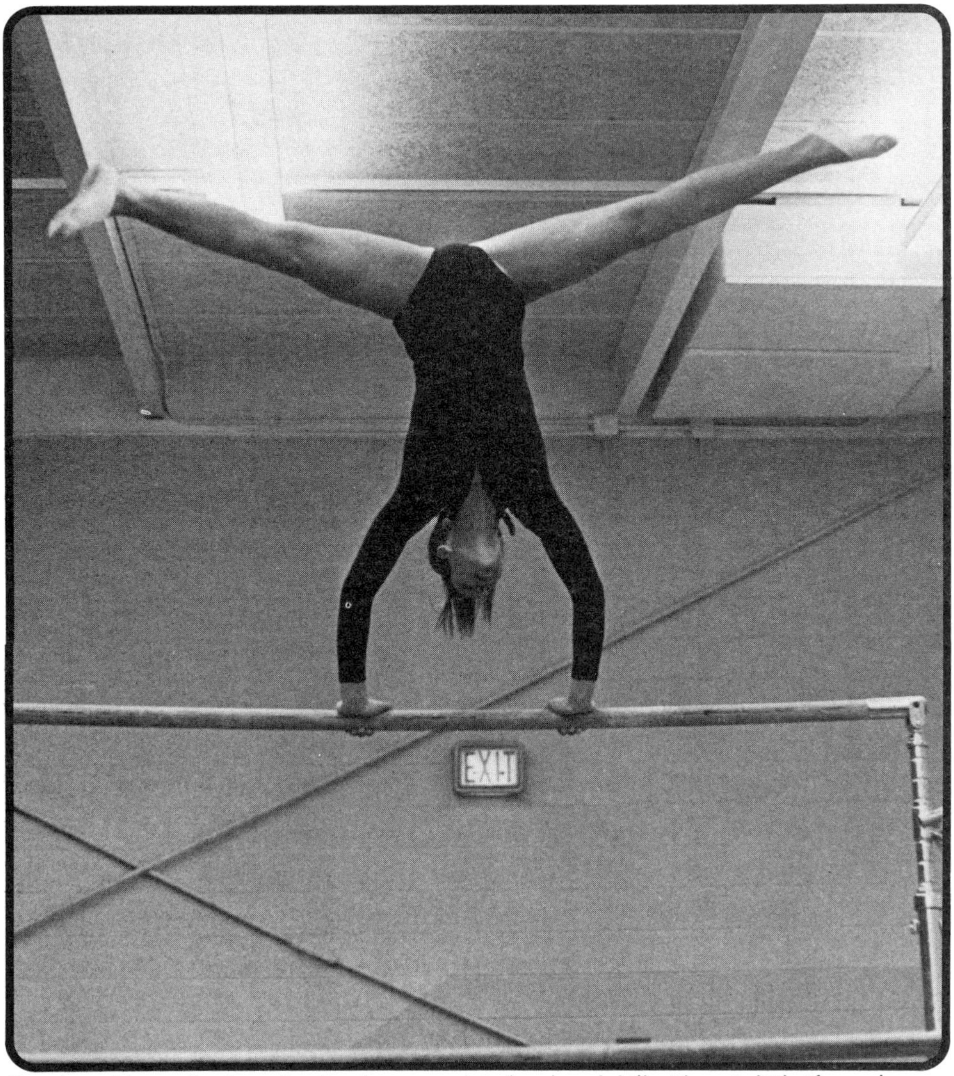

Practice with emphasis on fixation is appropriate for closed skills. There is little if any change from one attempt at performance to the next.

Habituate movements where critical cues are identical

goal are one and the same. That is the goal is to move in a certain way. The outcome, the number of points achieved, is directly tied to the movement. In other closed skills such as the basketball foul shot, the golf drive, the broad jump, or the flip turn in swimming, goal accomplishment is separate from the movement. In the basketball foul shot, for example, any one of several techniques or styles of shooting can be used without affecting the success rate of sinking the ball in the basket. Just think about the diversity in the movements used at the foul line by members of professional teams (there are certain movement principles that must be adhered to but a wide range of movements are possible). Still there is a distinct advantage to habituating or fixating the movement. For the basketball foul shot the basket is always the same height, the same distance from the foul line, in the center of the key, and the same diameter. The background may change, the players lined up at the key may be different but the critical cues are *always* the same and these are the cues to which movement should be habituated. A professional stepping up to the foul line assumes a consistent position, tries to place the body parts in the same relationship to one another as on previous attempts, holds the ball in precisely the same way, and attempts to move in the same manner as on other successful foul shots. In essence the performer tries to act like a foul shooting machine which has been finely tuned to the unchanging environmental cues associated with the foul shot. If the player succeeds, then the foul shot percentage will be high. In fact for most players the foul shooting percentages are higher than percentages from the floor. There are differences in each player from trial to trial, the pressures and anxiety induced by the game are different (imagine being fouled in the final seconds of the game with your team one point behind). The player who has fashioned himself into a foul shooting machine will be less affected by game pressures and fatigue than a player who has not achieved a similar high level of performance.

Think about the sports and skills listed below in relation to fixating the "perfect" movement. What cues in the environment remain constant? What aspects demand attention? What environmental cues affect the execution? What aspects of movement can be considered technique? What aspects can be considered personal style?

swimming dive
bowling
archery

track start
volleyball serve
field events (javelin throw, shot put)
tennis serve

In bowling, the position of the pins, the width of the alley, the distance to the foul line, the distance from the foul line to the pins, the weight of the ball, and the position of the arrows and dots remain constant. The initial position on the alley should be the same distance from the foul line, the same distance in relation to the right side of the approach, and in the same relationship to the pins, spots, or arrows as in other successful deliveries. The cues of the ball return, the back of the approach, the foul line, the dots or arrows, and the gutters might help the performer remain oriented in space and moving in the right direction. Technique may include such things as following through in the direction of the pins, keeping the arm close to the body on the forward swing, and releasing the ball close to the alley. Style may include the number of steps in the delivery, the grip on the ball, the method of releasing the ball, and the height of the backswing.

Diversification = change

Practice which emphasizes diversification is appropriate for skills in which the environment changes from trial to trial and in which objects and people move during each trial. These skills have been referred to as open skills. To do well at these skills the performer must have a repertoire of movements or be able to create movements which match the various environmental possibilities. In a tennis match, for instance, the ball may come to the forehand at a variety of heights, speeds, positions, and spins. If the forehand drive movement has been fixated through extensive practice with a machine that projected a ball at the same height and speed to the same court area each time the performer may be unable to successfully hit balls which come to different areas of the court at different speeds and different heights. In addition to being able to generate responses for various speeds, heights, directions, spins, it is necessary to differentiate among the various possibilities. When performers practice an open skill under "closed" conditions, they only see a particular combination of height, speed, and distance and do not learn to differentiate among different combinations nor do they practice the various responses that would match those possibilities. When learners practice an open skill under inappropriate fixated or closed skill conditions they will be handicapped when called upon to perform in the game environment. The game demands that players be able to discriminate

Inappropriate practice can negatively affect performance

different instances of time, space, and distance and that they develop appropriate motor responses to match the various environmental conditions.

Open skills require diversified practice to perfect the combination of variables and to abstract ideas about the relationship between input and response

Appropriate practice in an open environment includes several possibilities. In the beginning there should not be too many distinct possibilities presented. Perhaps three or four distinctly different situations might be used. The range of possibilities should be limited and as varied as possible so the learner will not have any difficulty recognizing their diversity. A ball might be projected to the player's forehand at fast, medium, and slow speed. These same speeds might then be projected to the player's backhand side. As an alternative a medium speed ball might be used and projected to the player's forehand, backhand, and center. Or the slow speed might be used and projected to the same places. In each instance the receiver would be informed about the range of possibilities so that he could plan accordingly. Following single variations of speed, distance, height, and direction, combinations of two variables, three variables, and all variables would be used. If, for example, there were only three possible speeds, three possible directions, three possible heights, and three possible distances the total number of possibilities which could be created are $3 \times 3 \times 3 \times 3$, a total of 81 different combinations. Imagine the combinations in an actual game! The purpose of varying the possibilities in a systematic way as illustrated is to assist the player in discriminating among the various combinations and to create responses to match the varying possibilities.

An abstract idea will enable the generation of responses for new input conditions

The diversification of practice and the use of different input combinations enable the player to develop an abstract idea about the relationship between input and response. What is the response that will lead to success under a particular set of input conditions? The formation of the abstract idea will enable the player to generate responses for input conditions that have not been previously presented.

The number of successive attempts at each particular combination is important to structuring practice for open skills. Should the player respond to each particular combination one, two, five, or ten times in a row? It seems clear that more than a single attempt is necessary so that the performer can use feedback from the previous attempt to correct errors before continuing. Ten trials may be too many because the performer begins to fixate.

In summary, the more open skills are practiced under game-like conditions, with the changing, unstable, unpre-

Repetition of responses are necessary to obtain feedback to guide successful responses

dictable possibilities, the easier it will be in the actual game. In fact this is also true in the case of closed skills because practice under game-like conditions means fixated, stable, and predictable events which should lead to habituated movements.

Identify some variables that change to produce different conditions for the following:

baseball batting
fielding a ball
blocking a spike in volleyball
rebounding in basketball
taking a lay-up shot in basketball
returning a tennis shot

When returning a tennis shot, the following variables must be considered: speed; direction; height; spin; angle; distance. Each of these variables can vary through an infinite range to produce many, many, different possibilities. It has been suggested that there are perhaps more than 1000 different sets of cues. To succeed the player must be able to generate a response to match each combination.

CHAPTER FIVE

achievement EVALUATION

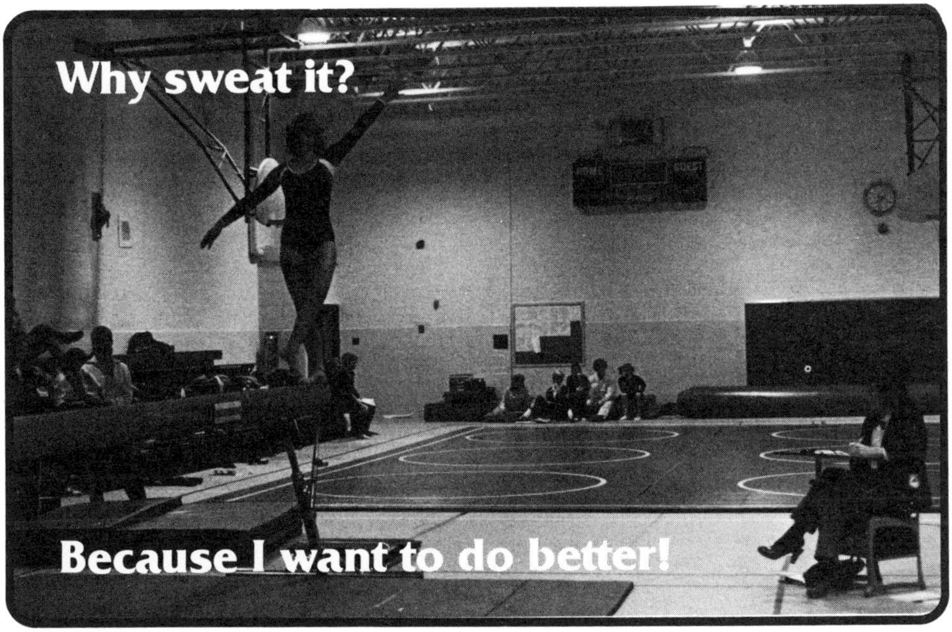

Photograph by Carlyjane Dunn Rice

What Do You Have To Help Me?

Improvement requires evaluation

A very important aspect of getting better is being aware of performance improvement. To track improvement and to uncover what requires emphasis in practice, it is necessary to evaluate performance. Before evaluation can occur, however, performance must be measured. When performance is measured a number is assigned to that performance. This number is called a score. In a gymnastics balance beam routine a 9.3 may be assigned as the score for a particular performance, a 9.7 to another, and a 9.95 to a third. These numbers represent the performance but they also indicate that, according to the judges, the third individual performed better than the second, and the second better than the first. Measurement can also be used to represent the performance of a single individual. A person who plays golf may have scores of 62, 55, 63, 54, 56, and 58 for nine holes in six consecutive visits to the golf course. The performance of this individual fluctuates but only within nine strokes. In addition the average number of shots taken for the first three visits is 60 while the average for the second three visits is 56 strokes. Measurement has revealed that the student has improved or evaluation and interpretation of the measurements taken have concluded that improvement has occurred.

These two examples are different. In the gymnastics example the score represented the movement process—how fluid, how graceful, how difficult, how error free was the performance. In the golf example the final stroke count represented the outcome or the result of the performer's movement. The performer moved to hit the ball but the concern is on the outcome rather than the movement. The number of total strokes is a reflection of the performer's movement but is not a direct measure of that movement in the same way that the gymnastics score is a direct representation.

By measuring and quantifying the movement itself or the outcome as appropriate to the type of skill to be learned, performance can be evaluated and progress assessed. It is important to evaluate performance and assess progress for a number of reasons:

- it maintains or heightens motivation, i.e., it keeps you going;
- it enables teachers and learners to assess the practice techniques being used;
- it permits evaluation of effort on the part of the student;
- it enables instruction sessions to be individualized for the students' needs and achievement level;
- it enables teachers to evaluate instructional methods;
- it focuses attention on the students' practice or instructional needs.

There are many specific ways of evaluating performance. They can be grouped into two general categories: measures which focus on the movement or the process of moving; measures which focus on the result or outcome of movement. Although this section focuses mostly on the *results* of movement a few comments about measuring the process of movement are relevant.

Performance process and outcome are measureable

When individuals watch a performer they may comment on the performance or the movement by saying, "Barbara is fun to watch, she moves effortlessly and smoothly," or "Wayne's form on the jump shot is textbook perfect," or "Valerie's form on the javelin throw is classic," or "John's groundstroke technique is faultless." Each of these phrases focuses on the individual's movement process, how he or she *moved*, rather than the outcome of the movement. The concern is not whether the ball went through the hoop, the tennis ball went over the net, or the javelin traveled a long distance. The focus is on *how the performer looked*. In the skills mentioned above, form or style of movement is not generally considered to be a requirement for success as long as the performer does not violate biomechanical laws which govern efficient and effective movement. There are skills, however, in which the quality of performance, the movement execution, is precisely what is measured. In competitive gymnastics, diving, and figure skating, points are awarded for movement quality. The judges in these events assign or subtract points according to an elaborate system which considers the degree of movement difficulty, the type of movement, aesthetic quality of the total performance, and style of the total performance. These systems are very elaborate and cumbersome and cannot easily be used by the performer to judge his or her own performance. Therefore we will consider performance outcome measures that can be used to compare different performances.

Performances can be compared with past self-performance or with others of the same age and sex

It is possible to compare a person's performance to that of others of similar age and sex. However since each individual learns at his own pace it is better to compare present performance to past performance.

Performance variables may be accuracy, distance, space, time, height, and weight

Commonly, performance is measured by assessing the outcome of movement in one or more aspects: accuracy; distance; speed; time; height; weight. All of these aspects are measurements of task accomplishment, i.e., to what degree did I accomplish the task. Some uses of these various aspects:

Accuracy

- batting average
- score in archery
- percentage of basketball shots
- pinfall in bowling
- percentage of first tennis serves in box

Distance

- how far you can jump
- how far you can throw the javelin
- how far you can jog
- how far you can throw a baseball

Speed

- how fast you can throw a ball*
- how fast your serve travels in tennis*
- how fast you can run

Time

- how long it takes you to run a mile
- how long it takes you to complete a specific task

Height

- how high you can pole vault
- how high you can jump

Weight

- how much weight you can lift

*This is difficult to measure directly but you can estimate the speed of a ball by dividing distance traveled by time.

What Else?

Another way of looking at skill performance requires that a number of task accomplishment measurements be taken, e.g., shooting percentages in basketball games during a season or part of a season and compared to find out how *consistent* performance is over the period of time involved. Does shooting percentage change drastically from game to game or does it remain relatively constant? Since basketball is a team game played against a variety of opponents some variation is to be expected. However a better player will be more consistent than a poorer player. Performance consistency can also be determined by calculating the standard deviation of performances — the calculation of this statistic is demonstrated in Table 5.1. The average performance can also be calculated over several games or over a season (the technique for accomplishing this is also demonstrated in Table 5.1).

What is a learning curve?

To obtain a clear picture of how performance may change from time to time and to evaluate learning, the change in performance, a performer might wish to plot a learning curve. A learning curve visually displays progress over time. The learning curve is a graph. On the horizontal or X-axis, plot time, attempts, games, or whatever unit of performance is to be measured. On the vertical or Y-axis, plot the task accomplishment score, shooting percentage, archery scores, or points awarded in a dive. In Table 5.2 Valerie's shooting

Table 5.1: Calculating the average and the standard deviation
(for illustration we will use Valerie's shooting percentages for 1978).

Game	%
1	35
2	37
3	43
4	45
5	40
6	50
7	48
8	52
9	55
10	60

Calculating the average

1) Add all the percentages
Sum = 465

2) Divide the sum by the number of games

$$\frac{\text{Sum}}{10} = \frac{465}{10} = 46.5$$

Therefore the average percentage of Valerie's shooting for 1978 was 46.5%. 1979 Average = 56.5.

Game	%	%
1	35	1225
2	37	1369
3	43	1849
4	45	2025
5	40	1600
6	50	2500
7	48	2304
8	52	2704
9	55	3025
10	60	3600

Calculating the standard deviation

1) Square each percentage (multiply it by itself)
(35) (35) = 1225
(37) (37) = 1369
......
......
......
(60) (60) = 3600

2) Sum all the squared percentages
22201

3) Square the average
(46.5) (46.5) = 2162.25

4) Divide the sum of the squared percentages by the number of games.

$$\frac{22201}{10} = 2220.1$$

5) Subtract the answer to 3 from answer to 4 and divide again by the number of games.

$$\frac{2220.1\text{-}2162.5}{10} = 5.785$$

6) Take the square root of the answer to 5 (what number times itself will equal 5.785?).
5.785 = 2.40

Therefore the standard deviation of Valerie's performance in 1978 was 2.40
1979 standard deviation = 2.34

Table 5.2: Valerie's shooting percentages for the first 10 games of 1978 and 1979.

Game	Percentages	
	1978	1979
1	35	43
2	37	50
3	43	56
4	45	48
5	40	58
6	50	62
7	48	55
8	52	60
9	55	65
10	60	68

Figure 5.1: Shooting percentages for Valerie during the first ten games of the 1978 and 1979 basketball seasons.

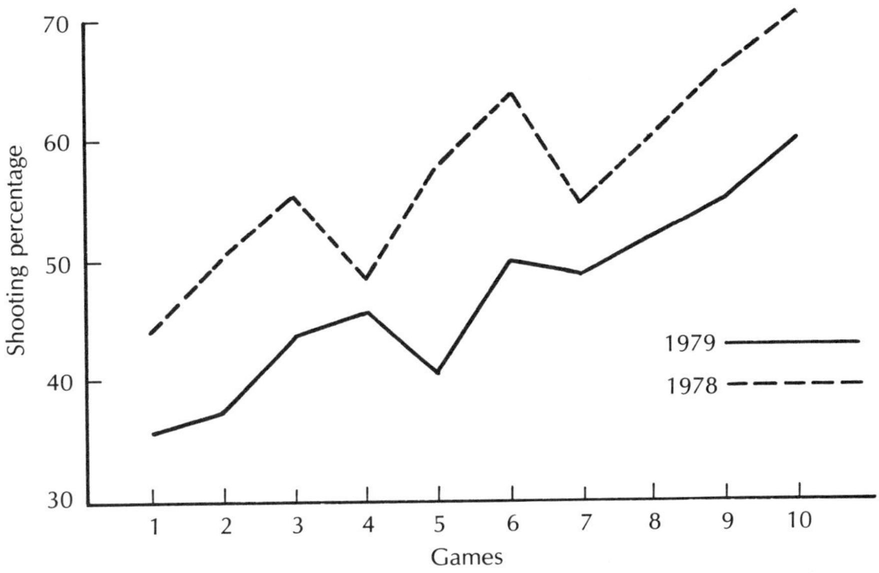

percentages for the first ten games of the 1978 and 1979 basketball seasons are listed. In Figure 5.1 these percentages have been plotted on a learning curve. It can be seen that Valerie made steady improvements in her performance during the first ten games of the 1978 season. How do these 1978 percentages compare with the percentages attained by Valerie during the first ten games of the 1979 season?

The graph indicates that Valerie improved her percentage over the first ten games of the 1979 season and that her 1979 percentages were better than those of 1978. In addition the graph seems to indicate that her performance is steadily and consistently increasing. Examine the learning curves shown in Figure 5.2. What skill is presented? When are measurements taken? What is measured? How many people are represented on the graph? What would you say about each person? How do they compare to one another? Why do you think they performed as they did?

The skill presented is the high jump and measurements are included for two members of the track team for eight meets in 1978. The measurement is the bar height for the best jump at each meet. Bob's performance seems to have worsened, since he jumped 5′5″ in the first meet of the season and only cleared a high of 4′8″ in the final meet. In addition Bob's performance demonstrates a steady downward trend. Dan, on the other hand, began the season with a best jump of 4′5″. When the last meet was over he had cleared a height of 5′8″. Responses such as motivation, amount of practice, distraction, physical condition, effort, commitment, and ability answer the question, "Why do you think they performed as they did?" While some of these reasons are plausible, the underlying causes cannot be analyzed without actually knowing the individuals being evaluated.

Adaptability is a mark of a skilled performer

Adaptability is another aspect of skilled performance which is related to evaluation. Adaptability is the ability to perform well under a wide variety of situations. Some individuals consider adaptability as *the* mark of a skilled performer. The term adaptability means that the shooting percentage of a basketball player is done equally well from many different areas of the court regardless of the type of defense used by the opponents. A tennis player who performs well with any type of equipment may be said to be more adaptable than one who cannot perform well with different equipment.

In assessing adaptability an individual's performances might be recorded according to the conditions under which the individual participates. For instance a high jumper might

Figure 5.2: Comparison of high jump performance for two track team members for the 1978 season.

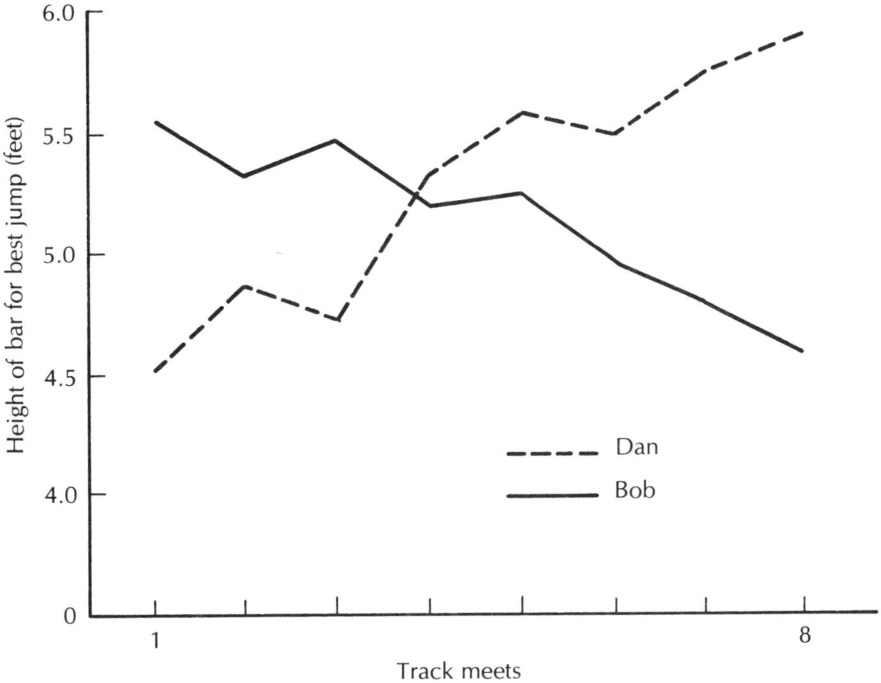

do extremely well in indoor meets but poorly in outdoor meets. He may do poorly in outdoor meets when the weather is wet but acceptably when it is dry. Another high jumper might do equally as well regardless of conditions. One basketball player might have high shooting percentages only in certain areas of the court while another player might have high percentages in all court areas. In each case the performer who does well under many conditions would be considered more adept than the performer who did well in a limited setting.

Summary

In evaluating skill performance:

- it is easiest to use measures of task accomplishment, e.g., accuracy, distance, speed;
- it is helpful to plot performance scores over time on a learning curve to see what progress or lack of progress is made;
- daily, monthly and yearly graphs can provide a good overall picture;
- summary statistics such as average performance or standard deviation of performance should be used to provide a meaningful evaluation;
- large increases or decreases in the learning curve should be explained;
- keep a record of performances under different conditions, like a shooting chart in basketball, to ascertain whether performance varies under different conditions.

The ability to focus on task accomplishment measurements will be helpful in utilizing feedback for performance improvement.

CHAPTER SIX

achievement

TIMING

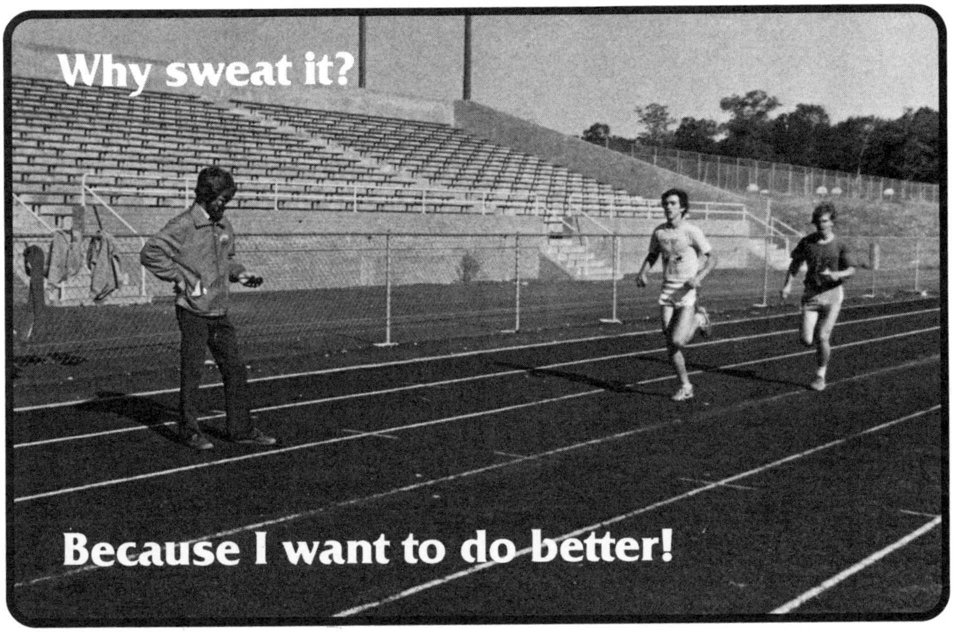

Photograph by Carlyjane Dunn Rice

What Do You Have To Help Me?

Closed skills timing depends on a coordinated sequented use of the necessary body parts

Superior athletes are often said to have "good timing." What does this mean? Is "good timing" responsible, even in part, for their superior performance? How can a performer develop good timing? Why is good timing important?

"Good timing" is a phrase often used to describe an athlete who has an extraordinary ability:

- to be in the right place at the right time;
- to be accurate in passing to moving teammates;
- to catch and hit moving objects with high accuracy;
- to coordinate and sequence the movements of various body parts.

To be successful at skill performance it is critical that:

- the body parts (hands, arms, feet, legs, trunk, and head) work together in a smooth, coordinated, sequential fashion;

Timing for open skills depends on coordinated body parts which match the time constraints imposed by the environment

- the timing of the execution of the total body movements match the time constraints imposed by the environment.

In closed skills, skills in which the environment is stationary, the first aspect is important; in open skills, skills in which the environment is moving, both are important. The ability to coordinate and sequence the timing of the body part actions in a consistent fashion is critical for successful movement execution. In the javelin throw, for example, coordinated, sequential action of the body parts will result in maximal distance, limited only by the individual's strength and angle of release. To assist a performer in improving performance of the javelin throw a teacher might evaluate the coordination and timing of the phases of the javelin throw: the preparatory phase; the first movement phase (the approach); the second movement phase (the release); the follow-through. A performer who completes the first movement phase and then pauses before initiating the second will lose the gained momentum. A performer whose approach is arhythmical and choppy will lose power. A performer whose arm/hand and leg/foot action are not coordinated with the body weight shift or the release will find that performance suffers. These aspects are related to the time course of the movement itself.

In the tennis forehand drive *both* the movement coordination and sequence *and* the matching of the movement to the time constraints imposed by the ball flight characteristics are important. The successful performer must initiate the forehand drive so that the preparatory phase (backswing) and the first movement phase (forward swing) occur prior to the arrival of the ball in the contact zone and the follow-through occurs following the contact. Thus the second movement phase, the contact, will occur coincidental with the arrival of the ball in the contact zone. In open skills the successful performer will be able to coordinate the movement execution as well as match the execution of that movement to the imposed environmental time constraints.

Why?

Timing is controlled internally and externally

The good timing, rhythm, and coordination necessary to successfully throw the javelin or to successfully hit a tennis ball are related to two different types of timing. *Internal timing*, the timing of movements so that each part of a jump shot,

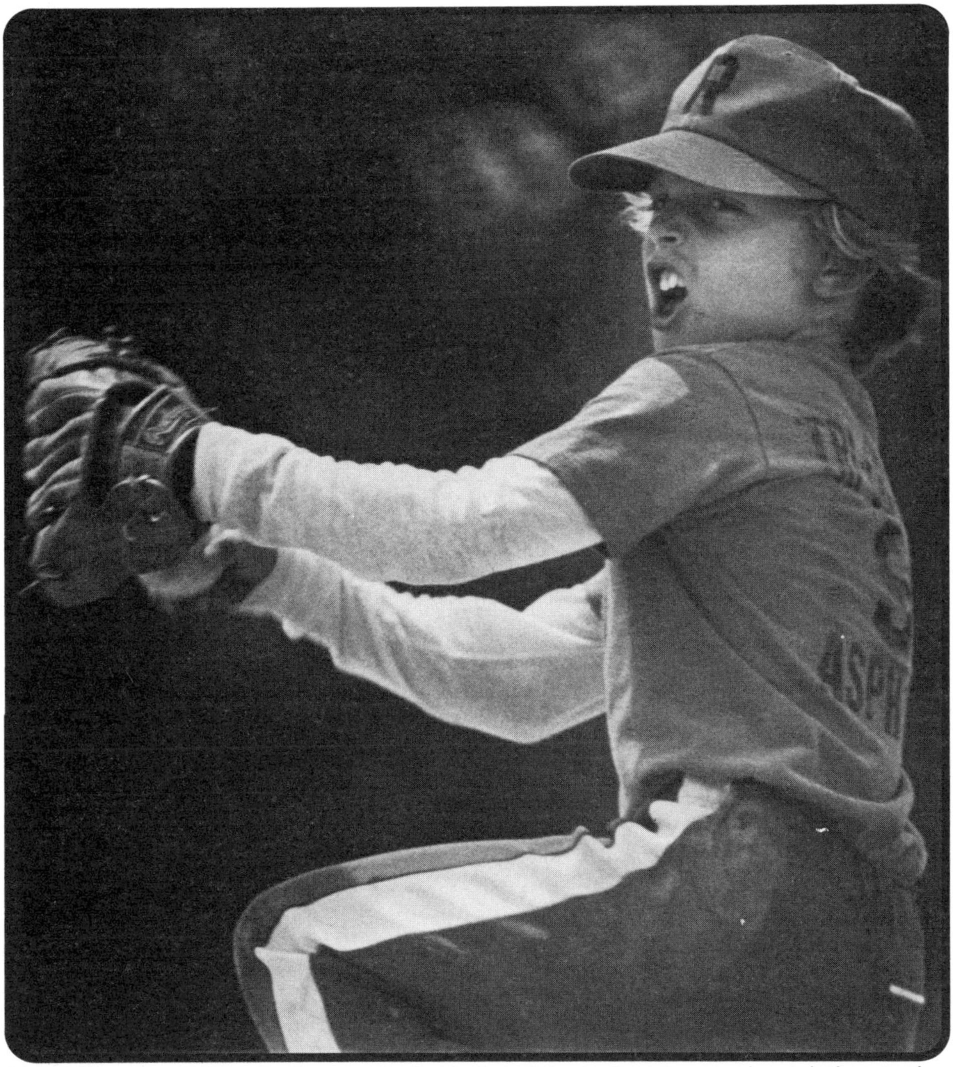

Photograph by Scott Forbes/Loudoun Times-Mirror

The ability to coordinate and sequence the timing of the body actions and match them to the environment in a consistent fashion is critical for successful movement execution.

for example, occurs at precisely the right instant in a controlled and coordinated sequence. *External timing*, the timing of the initiation (start) of your total movement, swinging the tennis racket, for example, so that the arrival of the racket head at the contact point coincides with the arrival of the tennis ball at a precise point and time (in the tennis example internal timing is also important).

Internal Timing

Skills are composed of sub-routines put together in proper time and space

Internal timing involves the ability to coordinate and regulate movements so that the various parts of the total movement follow in the correct timing and sequence. Sometimes it is helpful to think of the total movement of the tennis forehand drive as a whole made up of smaller parts. The whole tennis forehand drive is regulated by an executive plan and is made of small parts called sub-routines. The sub-routines for the tennis forehand drive may be listed as:

- grip;
- ready position;
- pivot, backswing, weight shift;
- forward swing, weight shift;
- contact;
- follow-through;
- return to ready position.

Practice leads to adjustments in the timing of sub-routine relationships

For the tennis forehand drive to be successful each of these sub-routines must occur in the proper sequence and rhythm (timing). If a player swings the racket back and does not pivot, the potential range of motion and the power to be gained from a longer swing distance will be lost. If the weight is shifted before or after the forward swing rather than with it, the extra power provided by your body weight will be lost. Every well-learned skill was once a set of individual sub-routines which were put together into a particular sequence. The sub-routines are poorly sequenced early in learning. With practice the sequence of the parts becomes established and the performance of each sub-routine becomes more automatic. Continued practice leads to adjustments in the timing of or the interrelationships among the sub-routines so that each part is initiated in relation to those sub-routines that have gone before and those sub-routines that will follow. Eventually the parts of the forehand drive become integrated into a single whole and the forehand drive is executed as a single unit with little or no attention to the parts or the interpart timing. At the same time, control of the execution of the tennis forehand drive passes from conscious attention to subconscious control.

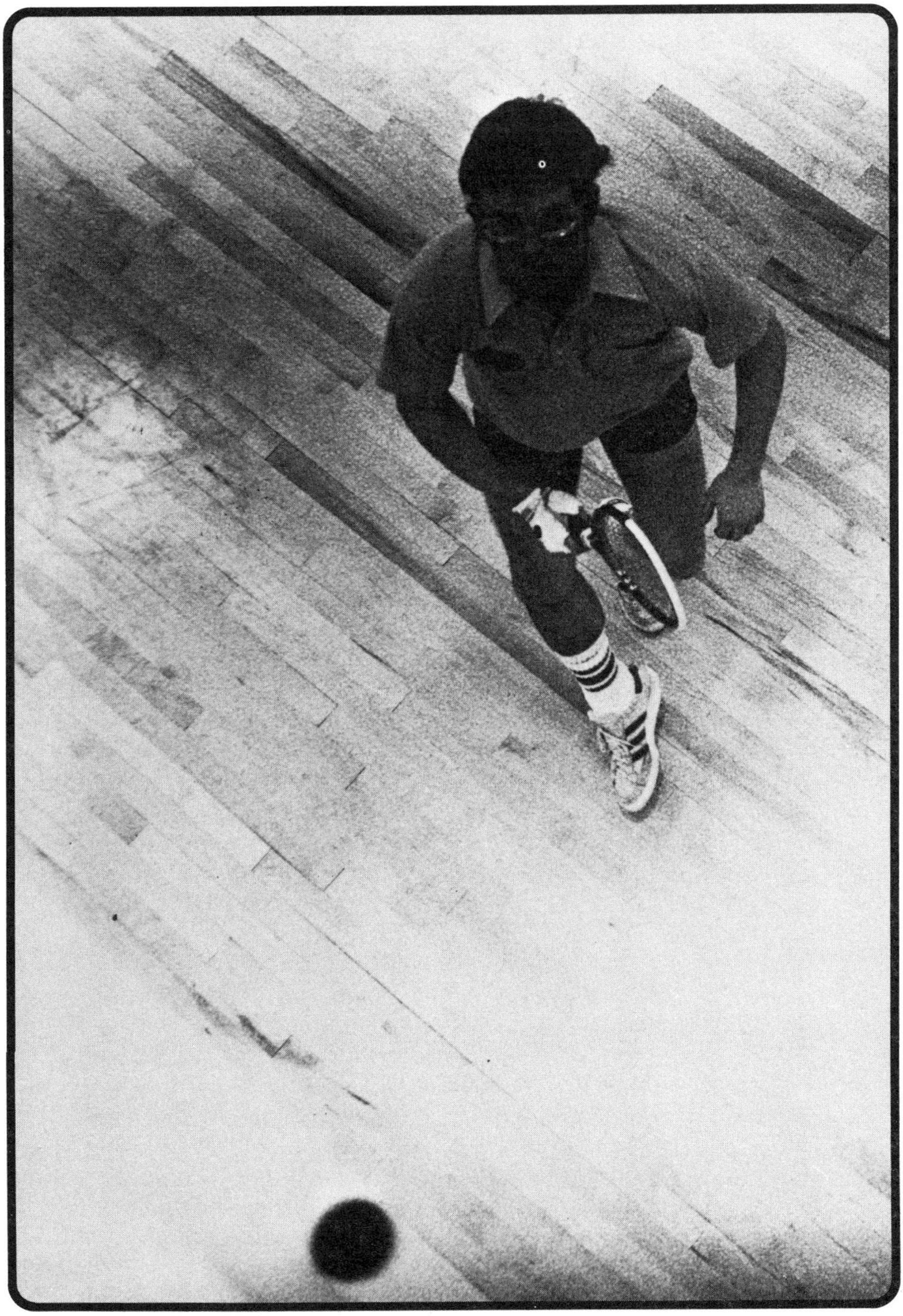

Photograph by Kit Brundage

Internal timing involves the ability to coordinate and regulate movements so that the various parts of the total movement follow in the correct timing and sequence.

At the same time the player is learning the forehand drive and establishing sequence, timing, and automatic control, he is also doing the same with the backhand drive, the serve, the lob, the volley, and other strokes. As he gradually becomes more skilled his conscious effort is focused on selecting the type of shot to use rather than the sequence and timing of a particular shot's execution.

Skill learning goes through three stages: cognitive; practice; automatic

It is believed that in becoming skilled the learner goes through three stages or phases: the cognitive phase; the practice phase; the automatic phase. These phases may be partially differentiated according to the internal timing ideas just presented. In the initial or *cognitive phase*, the sub-routines are selected and then sequenced in what seems to be the appropriate order discarding some sub-routines that don't seem to fit the situation and trying other sub-routines and sequences. Finally the learner is satisfied that the sub-routines selected are the ones that are most appropriate to accomplish the goal.

In the next phase the *practice phase*, the sub-routines are polished in execution and gradually integrated and interrelated and the timing of the sequence is refined. The learner begins to execute portions of the sequence without conscious attention thus releasing him to plan other things, like overall strategy or the next shot.

In the automatic phase, performance becomes independent of attention demands and the skill truly becomes a sub-routine within a larger whole of the tennis game. For an illustration of the hierarchial nature of sub-routines and executive plans see Table 6.1.

External Timing

The second type of timing requiring consideration is "external timing." External timing refers to the ability to initiate and execute a skill such as the tennis forehand drive so that the racket and the ball arrive at the contact point at the same exact moment. If the racket arrives ahead of the ball it is "early" and the ball will travel to the right (if you are right handed); if the racket arrives after the ball it is "late" and the ball will travel to the left (if you are right handed). It is also possible that the timing of the swing will result in the racket arriving so early or so late that it will miss the ball entirely. The effect of being early or late in relation to the contact point is illustrated in Figure 6.1.

Simply stated, external timing is the ability to anticipate the arrival of a ball and to regulate the initiation of a movement so

Table 6.1 Executive Plans and Sub-routines in Racket Games — Hierarchical Illustration.*

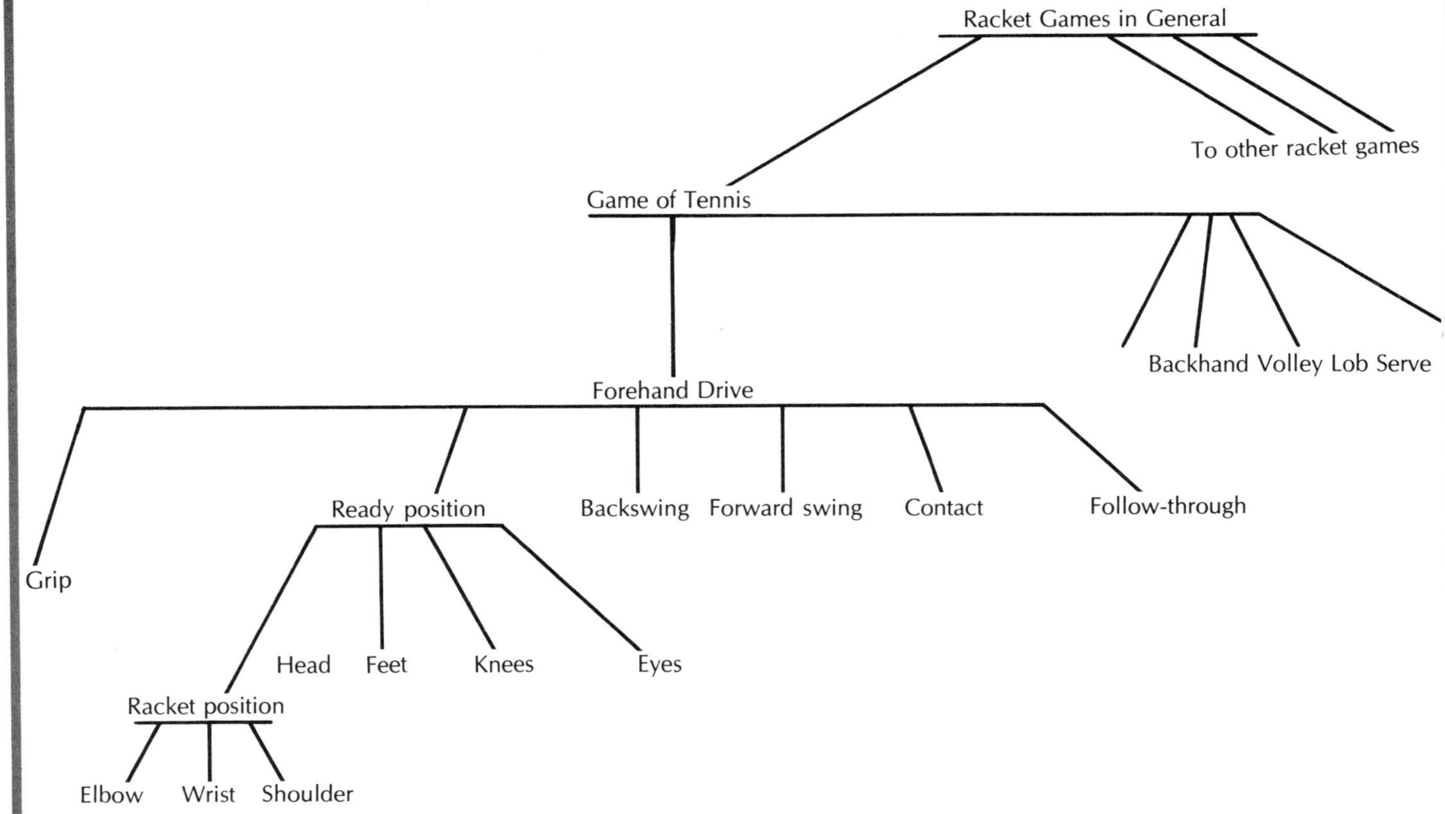

*adopted from Marlenuik, R. *Information Processing in Motor Skills,* Holt, Rinehart, Winston, 1976.

that in tennis, for example, the racket arrives at the contact point at the same time that the ball arrives at the contact point. There are several important aspects to be considered to be accurate and so exhibit good external timing. The player must:

- decide which direction the ball is moving;
- determine how fast the ball is traveling;
- decide when the ball will arrive at the contact point;
- decide where the contact point will be;
- decide what skill to use;
- move to the place where the ball will arrive;
- decide when to start the action so that he will be "on time."

When to initiate the skill execution so that the racket will arrive at the contact point "on time" requires that the movement begin one reaction time, and one movement time before the ball gets to the contact point. It takes time to move to the contact point and sufficient time must be left to get there (as in catching a ball). This last is not the critical problem, however, since a catcher can arrive ahead of the ball and be successful. The hitter in tennis cannot, in contrast, swing the racket and stop at the contact point to wait for the ball to hit the racket but must start the swing so the racket moves through the contact point and meets the ball in course (this technique is used to good advantage in bunting and the tennis volley but the ball does not have much speed or force and placement of these shots is critical for success).

Why?

External timing is affected by ability to discriminate the object from the background, speed plans, reaction, and movement time

There are a number of factors that affect "external timing" ability. These factors affect external timing in two ways: if each factor is not successfully accomplished then the completed response will be less than perfect; if each of these factors use time then the more time it takes to complete each factor the less time left for the overall response and the more rushed the remaining phases must be until in the final analysis the completion of the response will be "late" with respect to the arrival of the object. The factors include:

- the ability to discriminate the object from the background;
- the ability to discriminate among objects moving at different speeds;
- the ability to quickly plan or select a movement to match the objects' path and speed;

Figure 6.1: The effect of swinging a) early, b) late, and c) on time.

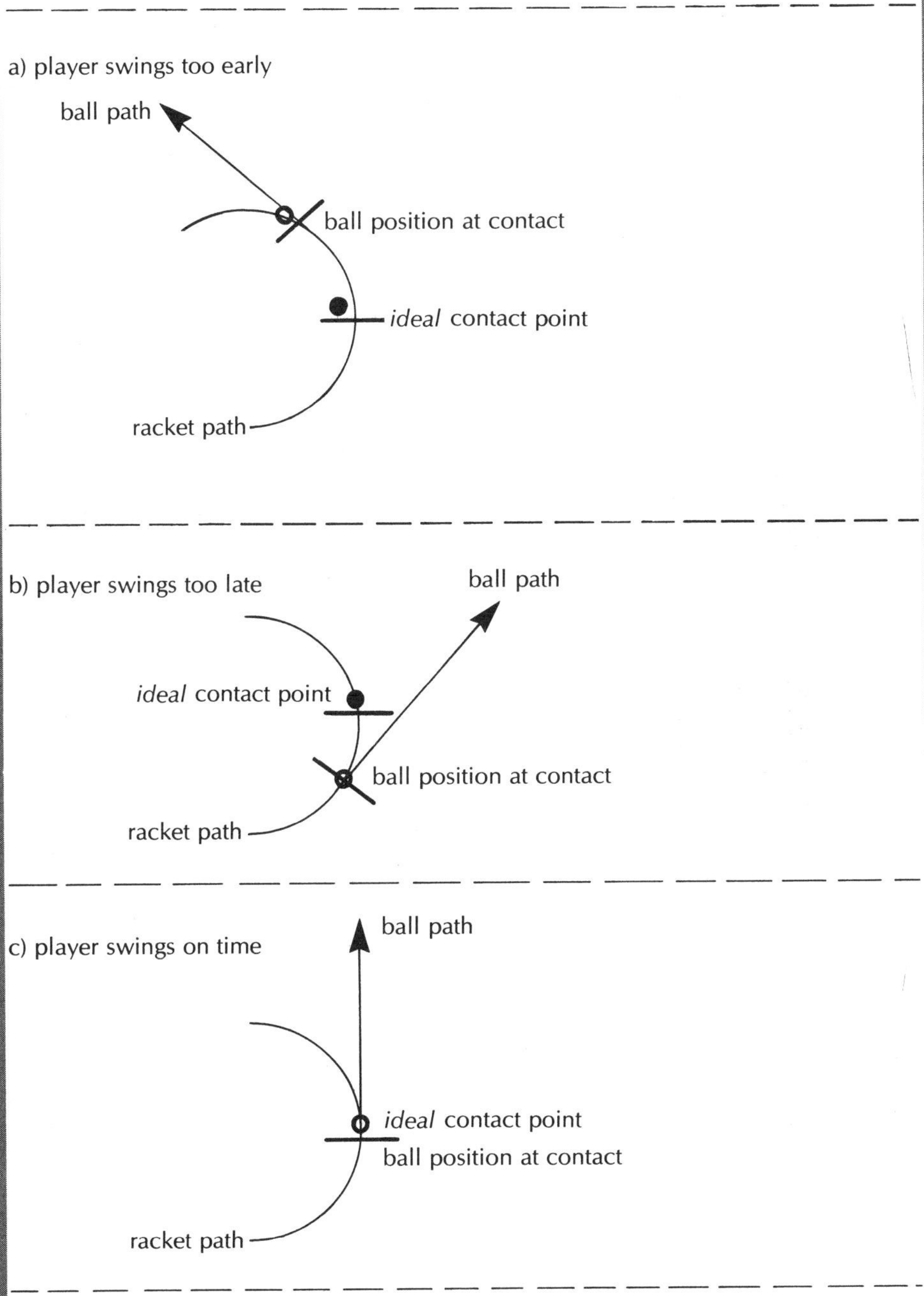

- reaction time;
- movement time.

Consider each of the factors in turn with special attention to improvement of each.

Discriminate object from background. The speed with which a performer can pick an object out of the background depends on characteristics of the person, of the environment, and the object. People vary in regard to the time it takes to extract objects from the background. Some people find it difficult and it takes them more time to pick out the object. Others find it easy and it takes them less time. The majority of people take an average amount of time. The ability to discriminate the object from the background can be improved in several ways:

What do you see?

- know what to look for;
- practice concentrating on the object by focusing on some barely discernable element of the object, e.g., the seams on a baseball, the dimples on a golf ball;
- make the object stand out more by painting it a bright color or by otherwise increasing the contrast between it and the background;
- change the background so it affords more contrast for the object;
- during early practice reduce the number of competing, irrelevant stimuli but gradually include them as practice continues;
- practice in many different contexts.

Discriminate among different objects and events. The ability to discriminate among objects traveling at different speeds, in different directions, at different angles, and such, is partly dependent upon individual characteristics and partly dependent upon object characteristics. It is helpful to think of each flight of an object as having a number of characteristics. These characteristics must be recognized and discriminated not only to successfully contact the ball but to be able to control the resulting flight of the ball. The ability to discriminate among different speeds, directions, angles and spins can be improved by:

- limiting the number of different speeds, directions, angles, and spins at first and varying only one element at a time then gradually increasing the number of characteristics which vary;

- learning to pick out the unintentional hints that an opponent gives with respect to how and where the ball will be hit;
- practicing at discriminating different object characteristics, e.g., standing behind the batting cage and watching the pitches.

Skilled performers select responses to fit a situation. Beginners create new responses

Quickly selecting the movement. This is the aspect of the chain of events that constitutes external timing that is most affected by practice and experience. Beginning players have to *create new responses* to fit situations; more advanced performers *select* the existing response that best meets the requirements of the situation. The notion of a schema as a rule that enables the quick generation of a response to fit a particular situation has relevance here. The beginner, for example, has no notion of the amount of force needed to throw a ball a given distance. He must as a consequence go through the process of deciding how much force will propel the ball a certain distance. After many attempts at throwing different distances the performer finally learns the rule, X force = X distance. This facilitates the quick generation of the appropriate force to throw any distance and this reduces the time taken by the response selection process. The best way to develop a schema is to vary the environmental conditions in which practice takes place, to practice in game-like situations, and to begin by varying a limited number of factors and gradually working up to a full range of factors.

What! You can't improve reaction time!

Reaction time and movement time. Of all the factors instrumental in external timing, reaction time is the only one that cannot be improved or changed with practice although minimal changes do take place with age. That is children under 10 and adults over 60 generally have slower reaction times than individuals between the ages of 18 and 50. At any age, however, reaction time is fairly consistent. It is the time it takes to initiate a response to a signal. This value is consistent and must be accounted for in initiating the movement in response to an external object.

Ah! But you can improve movement time!

Movement time is the time it takes to move a certain distance. Moving the bat from the starting position to the contact point over the plate is a good example. Unlike reaction time movement time can be improved through:

- increasing the explosive power of muscles through exercise;

Figure 6.2: The relationship between decision time, reaction time and movement time, and successful hitting.

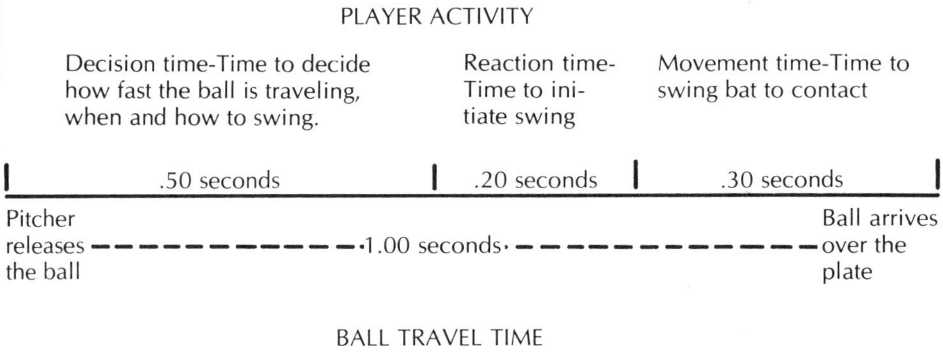

- decreasing the distance to be moved;
- shortening the length of the lever, e.g., choking up on the bat.

However, it's improvement in anticipation that really counts

The relationship between the factors identified and the speed of the object is illustrated in Figure 6.2. If it takes the ball 1.00 seconds to reach the plate and movement time is .30 seconds and reaction time .20 seconds then .50 seconds will be available for picking out the ball from the background, deciding how fast it is traveling, when it will arrive at the plate, and planning a swing before it *must* be started or be late. If it takes the ball 2.00 seconds to reach the plate then 1.5 seconds would remain to complete the other aspects. A response begun when the ball arrives at the plate will always be one reaction time and one movement time, or .50 seconds late. The response must be initiated .50 seconds *before* the ball reaches the contact zone.

Summary

Both internal and external timing are important for success in sport situations. Internal timing is important in all types of sports for smoothness and efficiency of movement and for generating maximal force with minimal effort. External timing is important in skills which take place in open environments because the performer must interact with moving objects and moving people to be successful. Development of external timing requires long hours of practice, under game or game-like conditions, making the types of judgments and decisions about moving objects and people that will occur in competition. A performer must be able to locate the important moving object quickly and discriminate its speed from all other speeds before predicting when and where it will arrive so that an appropriate response can be selected or planned and initiated. Some of the practice techniques suggested for open skills (in a previous chapter) are appropriate for developing external timing.

CHAPTER SEVEN

achievement

FEEDBACK

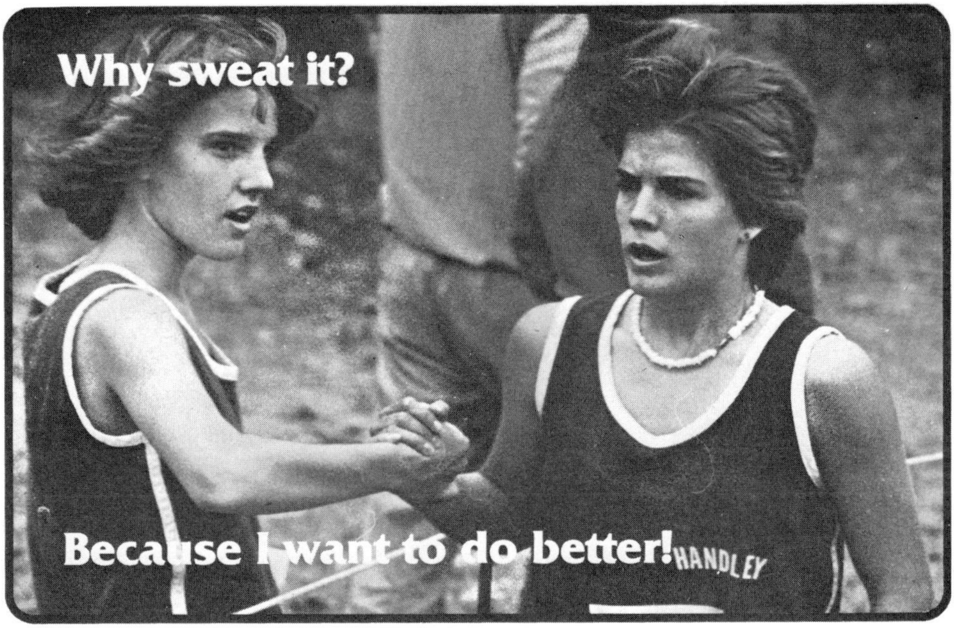

Photograph by Scott Forbes/Loudoun Times-Mirror

What Do You Have To Help Me?

Feedback is knowledge of results and knowledge of performance

Information about the outcome of performance and about the movement itself is absolutely necessary for performance to improve. This information is called feedback. Feedback provides information about the movement (kinesthetic feedback or knowledge of performance) and about the effects of that movement on the environment (knowledge of results). In actuality both types of feedback are received each time you perform. If it were possible to remove *all* available feedback, both knowledge of performance (KP) and knowledge of results (KR), learning would not occur. Feedback is important because it helps the learner decide what to do differently the next time. However there are ways to use it most effectively. For illustration purposes let us use a simple skill, tossing a ball underhand at a target.

Feedback directs adjustments in performance

The performer should stand about four feet from a four-ring target placed on a wall and toss the ball underhand aiming for the target center. For discussion purposes let us develop a sample performance. Although the actual performance may be different from the one we describe, it will probably proceed in a similar fashion. The first ball thrown lands short of the target and hits the floor. Performance is evaluated and it is concluded that the ball was not thrown hard enough. The next time the throw is more forceful but the ball is too high and hits the wall over the target. The conclusion is that the ball was thrown too hard. On the next toss "medium force" is used. This throw hits the wall directly below the target. In evaluating the three throws it is decided that the force is appropriate but that the ball must be released at a different point. The point of release problem is evaluated: if the ball is released too early it will travel downward and hit the floor; if it is released too late it will hit the wall above the target; if it is released at the correct point it will hit the target center.

After all the adjustments have been made the next throw lands on the target but at the outer right edge. On successive attempts both the release and the position of the body are adjusted until the balls land fairly consistently in the center of the target. The feedback from attempts to hit the target have been used to adjust motor performance by:

- attending to the ball's landing point;
- establishing what might have caused the ball to land where it did;
- adjusting the movement according to the decision above;
- executing the new movement and beginning again at (above) to evaluate it.

How?

Feedback involves movement and outcome information

To accomplish the changes in performance two kinds of feedback are required: feedback about the outcome of the movement; where it landed in relation to the target; feedback about the movement itself; what was done. In deciding what to do next the performer compares the outcome feedback with the desired outcome (goal), and the movement feedback with the planned movement. The relation between outcome and movement affects later behavior:

- if outcome matches the goal, and movement matches the plan then the performer is likely to throw the same way again;

- if outcome does not match but the movement does, then the performer is likely to try another plan after establishing what went wrong;
- if the outcome does match but the movement does not, the performer is likely to try the originally intended plan;
- if neither the outcome nor the movement match, then the planning process begins anew.

Resulting information is important in the accuracy development. It enables the performer to adjust the movement until both the outcome and the movement match with the intent. If outcome information is not available the performer may become more consistent, using the movement feedback, but will not become more accurate (it is not possible to eliminate movement feedback in an acceptable way, and most information on its importance is through research on neurological impairment).

Why?

Knowledge of performance is information provided by the nervous system about the movement. To use this information in adjusting performance the performer must determine whether the movement is the same as that which was intended. This requires the formulation of a plan of the movement prior to skill execution. Then after performance, the plan and the actual movement must be compared. Sometimes it helps to have someone else provide movement information to describe how the movement looked. However the individual's attention should be focused on certain specific aspects of the movement so that feedback is accurate, concise, and useable. In golf, for example, the wrist might turn outward at the top of the backswing; the club head might drop too far beyond the horizontal at the top of the backswing; the body might sway rather than twist during the backswing execution. An observer can help the performer work at keeping the club head horizontal by watching the angle of the shaft of the club in relation to the ground. After each set of shots the observer should pause a moment so the performer can analyze the movement. Then the observer should indicate whether the club shaft was beyond the horizontal or short of the horizontal. In time the performer should be able to make accurate judgements of the shaft position independently to correct the performance of the golf swing by "feeling" the angle of the club shaft. The performer becomes sensitized to what feels right and what feels wrong. It is important to try to remember how it "feels" when the angle of the club shaft is correct.

What Else?

Knowledge of results can also be used to evaluate performance. In executing the tennis forehand drive, for instance, the contact point and the path of the racket, and the angle of the racket face can often be determined by observing the flight of the ball (although most individuals consider knowledge of results to be where the ball lands; ball flight is in fact a result of the movement and can be very helpful since it is closer to the impact of the racket and ball). If the ball travels on a straight diagonal line to the right side of the court the player might have swung late or might have failed to pivot into position. If the ball travels on a straight diagonal line to the left of the court the player might be swinging early. If the ball consistently travels in a high arc when the intent is for it to travel in a straight, low line, just skimming the net, the racket face may be open as contact occurs; the grip may be incorrect or too loose or the racket head may be dropping on the swing. When teachers evaluate your performance and give hints on how to do better they often use outcome information to narrow down the possible errors. Performers can learn to do this for themselves by following the steps provided below.

- Know what to look for:
  where the ball goes out;
  how far the ball travels;
  what path does the ball take;
  what is the speed of the ball.
- Identify the things you might have done that could cause the error:
  held racket too loosely;
  swung racket in an arc;
  swung too early;
  swung too late;
  racket face was open;
  racket face was closed;
  failed to shift weight;
  led with the elbow;
  dropped the racket head.
- Link the performance error with the conditions in the environment right before you moved:

the flight of the ball;
the speed of the ball;
the feel of the racket.

- Decide how the response could or should be changed to reduce the error.
- Try to do the new response under the conditions in which the old response was done.
- Talk to yourself about the new response:
  "Grip the racket tighter;"
  "Swing through the ball;"
  "Keep the racket head up;"
  "Step into the ball;"
  "Follow through."
- Congratulate yourself for a response well done.
- Practice the new response under many different, appropriate conditions.
- Frequently assess the feedback from the body and the environment (performance information and outcome information respectively) to determine the status of improvement.

Why?

Finding out why you made a mistake. Information processing can be used to identify some of the problems that might lead to errors so that the adjustments referred to in the previous section can be made.

A mistake might have been made during the INPUT phase:

- examining the wrong area;
- looking at the right place but focusing on the wrong cues;
- focusing on the right cues but failing to discriminate direction, speed;
- discriminating direction, speed, but predicting the wrong place or time of arrival.

A mistake might have been made during the DECISION-MAKING phase:

- predicting correctly but choosing the wrong response;
- choosing the right response for the situation but not planning it properly.

A mistake might have been made in the OUTPUT phase (planning correctly but not performing the response as planned).

The first six errors can be called response selection errors. This is because they are related to improper attention to input or improper decision-making, both of which relate directly to the selection of the movement to be performed. The last error is called a response execution error. The correct response for the situation was selected but was not executed as planned. To utilize feedback to change the success rate the error cause must be first determined. It may be helpful to begin the evaluation of the movement and the outcome by answering the sequence of questions suggested in Table 7.1. After a bit of practice this sequence will become automatic and it will be done unconsciously.

Feedback comes from the situation or is added information

Types of feedback. There are several ways in which feedback can be classified as well as several means by which feedback can be administered. After reviewing the ways in which feedback can be classified and evaluating each in terms of its usefulness for learning we will focus on the usefulness of videotape replay as a means of providing information feedback. This is an important topic to consider since many people believe without proof that videotape replay is more effective than it actually is when it is used. For this reason individuals might be tempted to pay for its use at private instructional clinics, tennis centers, golf driving ranges, or may be tempted to take lessons from a professional because they use videotape replay.

Feedback can be given during or after performance

Feedback may be classified into that which is normally available versus that which is augmented or artificial. Feedback that is normally available is information that is inherent to the situation; it is always there unless specifically eliminated. Augmented feedback is added information. It is in addition to what would be ordinarily present in the situation. It is usually better to help the performer use the normally available information since it will always be there in the future. Often when augmented feedback is provided, performance improves. When it is removed, however, the performance gains may be lost. This loss may be lessened or prevented by using augmented feedback to provide information after the response has been made rather than during the response.

Feedback may be administered after the performance is completed or during the performance itself. Feedback provided while the individual is performing is called "concurrent" feedback. Feedback provided after the performance is labeled "terminal" feedback. There is always some concurrent feedback available. The sensations you get during movement provide information about movement speed, di-

Table 7.1 Performance analysis chart

Question	Answer	Action
1. Was the result of my movement successful?	YES	Repeat again
	NO	Go to 2
2. Did I move as I had planned?	NO	Try again
	DON'T KNOW	Try again, but decide how you intend to move and make a special effort to remember what you did or enlist outside aid.
	YES	Go to 3
3. Was I looking in the right place?	NO	Try again.
	DON'T KNOW	Ask someone where you should have directed your attention.
	YES	Go to 4
4. Was I focusing on the right cues?	NO	Decide what is important, and try again.
	DON'T KNOW	Get further information or be tested by someone.
	YES	Go to 5
5. Did I discriminate the cues properly?	NO	Practice noticing whether objects or people are moving at different speeds or are different heights, etc.
	DON'T KNOW	Get further information or be tested by someone.
	YES	Go to 6
6. Did I evaluate the cues properly?	NO	Practice estimating speed, height, time, etc.
	DON'T KNOW	Get further information or be tested by someone.
	YES	Go to 7
7. Did I choose the right response?	NO	What would have been more appropriate?
	DON'T KNOW	Ask someone what they would have done under the circumstances.
	YES	Go to 8
8. Did I plan my response properly with respect to timing, direction and sequence?	NO	Replan your response.
	DON'T KNOW	Review your plan with someone and ask for suggestions.
	YES	Go to 9

9. Begin at 1 (if you failed to achieve your goal, and the answers to questions 2-8 are all YES, ask for assistance in the evaluation process).

rection, and acceleration. Sometimes if a performance error is detected early in the sequence of movements it can be compensated for by adjustment of some aspect of the movement near the end of the sequence. For example if a bowler senses that the approach will end too far to the right, the path can be altered so that it will end where originally intended. It may also be possible to alter the ball release to compensate for an approach error.

Feedback may be combined

Normally available terminal feedback is also received. Some examples are volleyball (the ball going into the net or out of bounds on the serve), basketball (the ball going into the basket), and archery (the arrow hitting the target). This type of feedback, terminal feedback about the results of performance, is absolutely necessary for improvement. It is particularly useful when considered in combination with concurrent feedback. Information about the movement and information about the result of movement must be integrated to improve your performance.

Augmented terminal feedback is information provided by someone else or something else after performance. This is usually helpful if the performer is given the opportunity to evaluate and assess his own performance first and then use the additional information to check his impression. For example a coach or teammate might indicate that a player has been consistently falling away from the shot in basketball practice and in games or that a golfer has been lifting the head on the tee shot in golf. The performer may have surmised that these were possibilities by checking outcome errors but was not able to identify the precise problem. The extra feedback after performance (augmented terminal feedback) can help players to evaluate the cause of their error, and to plan future responses.

Which type of feedback is least effective

A type of feedback that has little if any lasting value in terms of performance is augmented concurrent feedback. Gains made when using this feedback are lost almost immediately upon its termination.* Some examples:

- devices that help groove the golf swing;
- auditory cues to help aiming;
- gloves or wearing apparel that remind players when they do something wrong;

---

*In the case of biofeedback, whose success might seem to belie this statement, the user is encouraged to identify some inner cue which can be used when the augmented concurrent feedback is no longer available. Unless this is done gains made will be lost.

- devices that indicate how much tension is being exerted;
- pacers that help a runner maintain a constant pace.

The individuals who employ these devices become dependent upon them to perform as required; once use is discontinued, performance regresses to previous levels.

Augmented terminal feedback is most effective

Feedback may be provided immediately or it may be delayed for a period of time. The distinction between these two is relevant only when augmented feedback is concerned (the human system operates on normally occurring delayed concurrent feedback; processing time, such as that indicated for reaction time, effectively delays all communications within the system; feedback about how you moved and about the outcome of your movement is always delayed). Since it has been demonstrated that augmented concurrent feedback is not very useful we need only be concerned with the manipulation of augmented terminal feedback. Should information be given to the performer immediately after the performance ends or should there be a delay? If a delay, how long should it be?

Why?

It is best to delay augmented terminal feedback briefly until the performer independently analyzes the performance. It is also useful for the performer to utilize the information provided in planning and executing another response as soon as possible. For example, information given to the individual about the performance in a game will not be as useful if the individual cannot have an opportunity to put the feedback into practice. In addition the player needs to have the opportunity to replay those situations about which feedback is administered.

Verbal feedback is more direct and inexpensive

Two other aspects of feedback are sometimes discussed. One relates to the mode of providing verbal or visual feedback. The other relates to whether the feedback should encompass a single attempt or a series of attempts. In considering the verbal versus visual choice, the cost of providing good visual feedback should be considered as well as the delay inherent in any type of visual feedback. Verbal feedback can be provided on the spot. The feedback can be given or accompanied by cue words that the performer can remember on the next attempt. It is inexpensive and can employ checklists or peer observations or both and requires virtually no equipment. The use of verbal feedback does have some drawbacks in that:

- an unskilled observer might miss some key points;
- there is no lasting record of the actual performance;
- it may not be as motivating as visual feedback although it may be equally informative.

It should be noted that effective use of visual feedback requires the concommitant use of verbal feedback to focus the performer's attention on relevant information.

Visual feedback will require verbal feedback to focus attention

The final consideration is whether feedback should be provided after every attempt or whether it should be based on numerous attempts. When the skill to be learned is simple, feedback after every trial is the quickest, most effective means of insuring rapid progress. With complex skills, however, it is often better to wait until the performer has made several attempts and then identify the most prevalent or serious error the performer is making. In complex skills the performer has many aspects to consider and so it is common for errors to vary somewhat from attempt to attempt. Therefore accumulated feedback can enable the observer to pick out the single critical error and focus the learner's attention on that, thus providing a single focal point for a new series of attempts.

Videotape replay. One means of providing feedback which is in common use in public as well as private organizations is videotape replay, often abbreviated VTR. Many ski areas, golf courses, racquetball clubs, tennis clubs, and the like have discovered that people want to excel quickly without the fuss and bother of tedious hours of practice. The easy accessibility and ever decreasing cost of VTR equipment coupled with the delight experienced by many people in "seeing themselves on TV" has led to the use of VTR as an enticement to "join our club, we provide VTR," "ski here, watch yourself improve on TV," "watch your swing on TV, then we show you how to improve it." It has been shown, however, that VTR when used improperly is no more effective for learning than usual instruction procedures. In addition when it is effective it is generally far less so than individuals would like to believe. Some guidelines for the effective use of VTR are presented in this section.

Verbal cues should be used in conjunction with videotape replay to direct the performer's attention to specific aspects of the performance that are important. Suggestions such as, "look at your racket face, it is open," "you stepped forward before you started your swing," "you tossed the ball too high," will assist the player in seeing those aspects of the picture that will help speed improvement. It will also provide a verbal statement that the performer can remember to cue behavior at a later time.

Isolated parts of performance may be viewed by using a camera with a zoom lens. This can be especially helpful when handling skills that require small movements or when highly skilled players require help with a particular portion of a skill. In archery the VTR operator may zoom in on the release hand of the archer; in basketball on the fingers of the release hand; in golf the hand position at the top of the backswing; in gymnastics the body position on a vault.

Practice following the administration of the VTR and after decisions are made about how the skill should be modified is crucial. When open skills are involved it would be helpful if the practice situation were recreated during the post-feedback practice. For example in a VTR of a particular play in football, the coach might point out an error that the players made in the pattern or direction of running and then might run that same play again so that the performance could be corrected. This same idea should be carried through in basketball, hockey, and soccer, as well as in tennis, badminton, etc.

Models of correct performance are sometimes useful in helping the player understand what is expected or required. Care should be taken, however, to focus on general aspects of movement in those activities where a specific form is not dictated by the rules. In tennis, for example, the viewer's attention might be focused on the model's weight shift, following the shot to the net, the relationship between the initiation of the swing and the weight shift rather than on particular aspects of the way the individual moves. In skills that demand adherence to specific form, e.g., diving, ice skating, gymnastics, information in regard to a particular movement pattern would be perfectly appropriate.

Both objective and subjective viewing of video-replays are needed

The number of times that VTR is administered is important. The critical number seems to be five. It is preferable to have multiple viewing at each of the five sessions in which VTR is used. It has been suggested that the VTR system at the Montreal Olympic Games in 1976 may have operated to the advantage of those performers who saw themselves more frequently (this is unlikely since Olympic caliber performers require much more specific feedback than VTR can provide).

The focus of VTR should be shifted to provide attention to other aspects or views of the same performance. This can be seen in the replays sometimes shown in televised football or basketball games. When the viewing angle changes, the interpretation of the event sometimes changes. In the instructional use of VTR two principal views are used, the objective view in which the performer sees himself or herself as others would, and the subjective view, the view you see from your position.

What should the replay show?

The final point is that information provided should be *goal consistent*. That is, in diving, where the performer is rated on the movement, the VTR should focus on the movement. In tennis where the goal is to get the ball over the net in a way which prevents the opponent from returning it, the VTR should focus on the total situation. At the very least both views should be available.

It should be noted that the suggestions provided for VTR

- verbal cues,
- practice following feedback,
- use of models,
- attention to isolated aspects of performance,
- number of administrators,
- focus and feedback, and
- goal consistency

are also relevant for other feedback modes. Attention to these aspects can increase the effectiveness of all types of feedback.

CHAPTER EIGHT

achievement

CHANGE

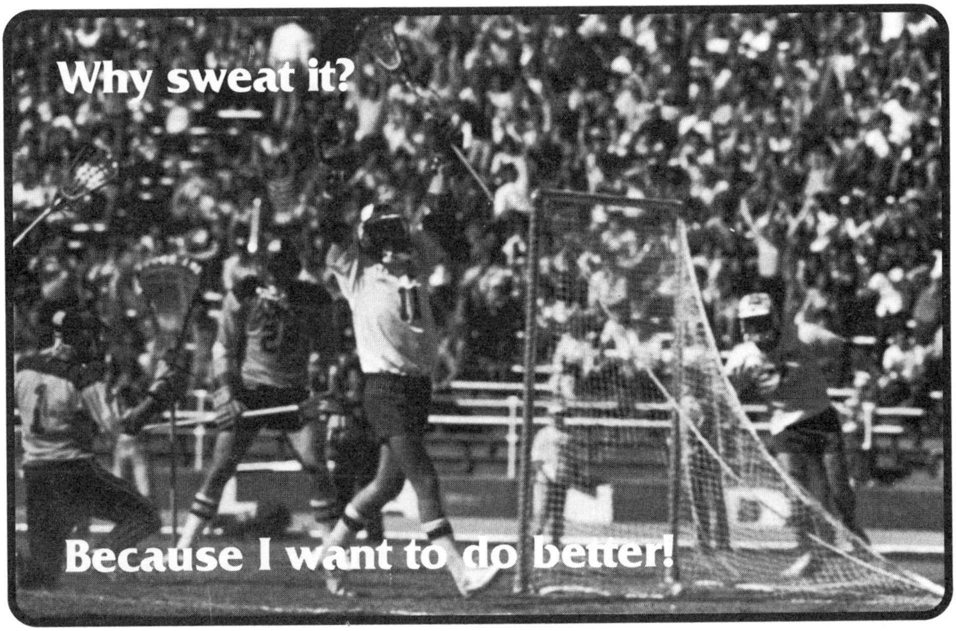

What Do You Have To Help Me?

Performance improves in accuracy, consistency, control, coordination, adaptibility, deliberativeness, and planning

Motor skill performance improves as the result of changes that take place in INPUT, DECISION-MAKING, OUTPUT, and FEEDBACK operations. As a result of these changes in information processing the performer and/or the performance will be:

- more accurate;
- more consistent;
- more coordinated;
- more controlled;
- more adaptable;
- more deliberate;
- better planned.

More *accuracy* results when performance results are closer to the goal.

More consistency results when the outcome of performance is less variable, the set of outcomes achieved is more alike, the scores are closer together. Performance can become more consistent without becoming more accurate. In fact once performance becomes more consistent it is easier to gain accuracy.

More *coordinated* performance results when the body parts involved in the skill performance become better synchronized in time and space. This results in more efficient and effective performance.

More *controlled* performance results when the amount of effort used to execute the skill is appropriate to the task. The golfer who taps the putt just hard enough to sink it is using more controlled effort.

Performance is more *adaptable* when the performer can respond effectively under a wide variety of conditions. The tennis player who can effectively return tennis ball hits at various speeds, heights, directions, and spins is demonstrating adaptability.

Performance will be more *deliberate* because the performer will not need to rush to interpret the event, plan a response, and initiate it at the last minute. Rather the performer will be able to base interpretation and response choice on early cues (cue abbreviation) and will thus appear unhurried in the performance. The tennis player who slowly and deliberately moves into hitting position, establishes a base, then executes the appropriate response is more deliberate than the player who seems frenzied and rushes to hit the ball on the run and always appears to be arriving at the last minute.

Finally as skill increases, the performer does not have to attend as closely to the input, decision-making, and response phases. Thus the player is free to focus on short and long range strategy which will lead to the performance appearing better *planned* with the advanced players in better control of the game or play.

These observable improvements are the result of changes in the ability to process information and in the method of processing information. Individuals have recently become interested in how the processing of information changes as learning occurs. If we know how information processing changes then we may be able to plan practices that will speed these changes. If we know, for example, that more advanced performers focus attention on relevant stimuli in the environment while beginners tend to look at irrelevant stimuli, then we might use some method of making important stimuli "stand out" to force the beginner to attend them.

The major changes that take place in the ability to process information may be categorized under the broad headings used earlier: INPUT, DECISION-MAKING, OUTPUT, and FEEDBACK. These changes are:

- performers learn where to look;
- performers learn what to look at;
- performers spend less time absorbing information;
- performers learn to differentiate relevant (important) and irrelevant (unimportant) information;
- performers learn to predict the outcome from a few early cues;
- performers can discount (eliminate) certain outcomes as being improbable or less probable than others;
- performers begin to process "sets", or patterns of stimuli rather than individual stimuli;
- performers develop verbal labels for the patterns of stimuli that are characteristic in their sport;
- performers can integrate information from several important sources;
- performers have a highly developed notion of movements to match environmental events;
- performers can quickly select appropriate movements;
- performers can respond to events that are novel;
- performers can automatically execute movement segments;
- performers can integrate the separate aspects of movement;
- performers are more adaptable and able to perform successfully under a wider variety of conditions;
- performers' attention shifts from the short range consideration of "this shot" to consideration of overall strategy for the long range aspect of "this game" or "this rally" or "this play";
- performers can guide their own learning through use of available feedback;
- performers can evaluate their own performance through use of internal systems.

Why?

As learning occurs and players become more skilled these changes in information processing lead to quicker, more accurate, more consistent performance. To provide some notion of how practice might be structured to speed changes, each of the broad segments of information processing will be considered: INPUT; DECISION-MAKING; OUTPUT; FEEDBACK. It should be noted that improvement in each of the broad segments is necessary but not sufficient for improvement in overall performance since in the final analysis the whole of information processing must be integrated.

INPUT

The major factors related to improvement in the INPUT segment are:

- *orienting*--the ability to look in the right place;
- *selective attention*—the ability to concentrate on relevant stimuli and ignore irrelevant stimuli;
- *cue abbreviation* — the ability to predict the outcome on the basis of a few, early cues;
- *probability planning*—the awareness of the likelihood of various outcomes or events.

Previously the ENVIRONMENT has been identified as the source of INPUT. The ENVIRONMENT consists of *all* the external and internal cues affecting performance. Thus for a basketball player the environmental cues are among others:

external —

the court,
the stands,
the fans,
the referee,
the opposing players,
the teammates,
the coach, and
the distance to the basket;

internal —

fatigue level,
anxiety level,
pain, and
distracting thoughts.

What would be included in a list for a football player? for a swimmer? for a gymnast? for a tennis player at the U.S. Open?

It is helpful to think of the environment as consisting of sections. Some sections contain information that is important (relevant) to the planning or selecting of a response while other sections contain only unimportant (irrelevant) information. This unimportant information may be thought of as distracting because it takes the player's attention and concentration away from the important information. Since much of the information that we receive from the environment is visual let us consider orienting with respect to the eyes.

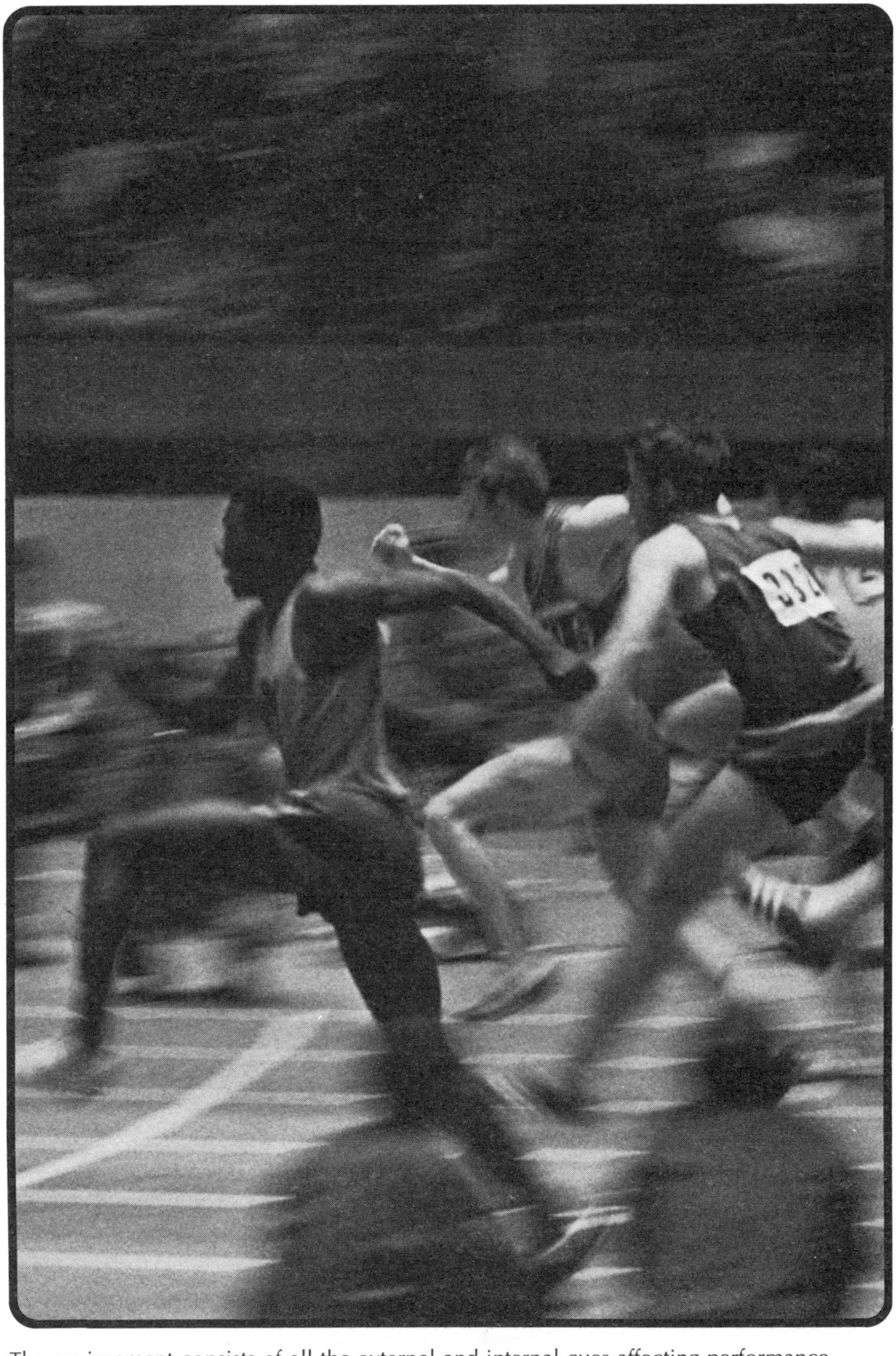

Photograph by Courtesy Scholastic Photography

The environment consists of all the external and internal cues affecting performance.

Orienting. The performer must orient or turn the eyes toward that section of the ENVIRONMENT that contains the most important information. This response may be thought of as the response the player makes to the question "Where should I look for the information I need to plan my response?" Beginners usually don't have any idea where to look and teachers rarely provide any clues about where the important information is to be found.

Orienting to the most important information is important to success

Orienting to the section of the environment which contains the important information is the first step to achieving success since the performer must create or select a movement which is matched to the environment in which it is performed. If the performer is not looking in the right section, at the section in which this important information is to be found, then he will not "see" this information. There are several factors that will affect success in orienting to the correct portion of the environment:

- the familiarity of the background;
- the size of the peripheral, visual field;
- past experience;
- verbal cues from others;
- the intensity of unimportant cues.

Experience and skill help trigger orienting responses

As individuals become more skilled through past experience, cues in the environment trigger or set off the orienting response. For instance as the game develops the player expects that certain plays will occur and "looks" for cues in the environment that these plays are happening. When this cue or these cues are detected the player immediately orients toward the section of the environment in which they are found and focuses on the information.

If the game occurs in a familiar setting such as the player's home court, the player will be better able to detect the cues which trigger the orienting response. This is because of the decreased likelihood of new and different background cues which will distract the performer's attention.

Beginners have a narrow peripheral field

The peripheral visual field can be described as narrow or broad. Having a narrow peripheral visual field is like gazing through a tunnel. One can only see what is directly in front of him. Having a broad peripheral visual field means that cues to the side of the head can be detected when the player is looking straight ahead. The size of the peripheral visual field is affected by:

- stress level;
- the complexity of the environment;

- the level of difficulty of the skill;
- the degree of uncertainty of events.

As each of these increases, the size of the peripheral visual field decreases. For beginners each of these factors is high; therefore beginners can be expected to have a narrow visual field. This results in an inability of beginners to detect and respond to cues which are not directly in front of them. As skills increases, these factors decrease so that size of the peripheral visual field increases (it is important to note that some sports require that the performer purposefully narrow the focus of vision for better concentration; however, the beginner rarely has the luxury of choice since circumstances dictate the size of the peripheral field).

Verbal cues are helpful

Finally verbal cues from others will help the performer to shift visual focus to important sections of the environment. In basketball it is common to see and hear players signalling for the ball. In tennis it is common for teachers to tell beginners "watch the ball."

Helping the learner develop orienting ability

In assisting performers to orient to appropriate environmental sections, the coach or teacher might use any or all of the following:

- manipulate the familiarity, complexity, and uncertainty of the environment;
- manipulate the difficulty of the task or provide verbal cues about where to look, intensifying important cues;
- reduce the intensity of unimportant cues.

In addition watching games can help you develop a sense of where the action takes place on particular plays or in certain situations. If however the conditions under which practice occurs are manipulated to facilitate learning they should gradually be returned to normal as learning occurs. Otherwise the player will be unable to cope with the normal game environment.

Cues are important for planning or selecting successful responses

Selective attention. Orienting is the answer to the question "Where should I look?". Selective attention is the answer to the question "What should I look at?". Just as the total environment can be apportioned into sections which contain useful or important information and those which do not, so the cues themselves can be categorized into those which are important in relation to the response and those which are unimportant. As might be expected players with more skill and experience seem to instinctively know what is important. Well, for most of these players this knowledge is not "instinctive" but has been achieved through long tedious hours of practice under game conditions, in game situations, and even longer hours of watching the game. These players are learning to understand the regularities and predictabilities of the game they want to play. They learn that certain "cues" are present when certain responses are successful. They learn that certain cues are important to planning or selecting a response. Some factors which affect the ability to selectively attend to the important cues are:

- the contrast between the important and unimportant cues;
- the ratio between the important and unimportant cues;
- past experience;
- the intensity of the important cues.

Ability to discriminate cues is important to skill development

Before the learner can focus on the important cues he must be able to differentiate or discriminate them from the unimportant cues. This concerns contrast. When watching television try adjusting the contrast so that the entire picture becomes almost a single cue. Now gradually return the contrast to normal. Beginners are sometimes unable to tell the difference between what is important and what is unimportant; everything looks the same to them. Therefore it takes them much longer to make decisions about what to look at and they sometimes have to look at *everything* one or more times to decide.

Ability to differentiate events is a prerequisite to selectively attending these events

An interesting example of the ability to differentiate cues relates to different types of snow. Eskimos can differentiate 22 types of snow; that is they have 22 names for different types of snow conditions. How many kinds of snow can you identify? Typically cross country skiers are able to identify respective matching waxes to different types of snow. An agricultural specialist can identify many different types of soil, a geologist many different types of rocks, a skilled baseball batter many different types of pitches. *The ability to differentiate different events is a prerequisite to selectively attending to those events and this ability improves with practice.* The teacher or coach can assist the beginning player to discriminate among different cues by pointing out the crucial differences that the player should examine.

Some individuals are quicker at recognizing stimuli

Preventing the opponent from discriminating the important cues is a prevalent strategy in sport. In football the quarterback attempts to embed the signal to snap the ball in a string of numbers which vary in number and cadence. When the ball is snapped the offensive players attempt to "hide" the ball so that the defensive team members will not know who has the ball. What are other ways in which players attempt to camouflage their intent?

Some individuals are quicker at differentiating the important from the unimportant stimuli. This may be a result of past experience or it may be an inborn trait. However there are few people who are extremely good and few people who are extremely poor; most are average and can benefit from the use of

- verbal cues concerning what to look for,
- techniques for highlighting or increasing the intensity of the important cues, or
- advance warnings about what to expect.

Another aspect that is related to the ability to selectively attend important cues is the ratio between the important and unimportant cues. If there is a single important cue and 50 unimportant cues, finding the important cue may be like "finding a needle in a haystack." If there are ten important cues and only two unimportant cues the task will be much easier. Teachers and coaches should attempt to manipulate the ratio between important and unimportant cues for beginners so that the task will be easy at first and then gradually change the ratio until it is returned to normal.

Cue abbreviation is important to skilled performance

Cue abbreviation. The notion of cue abbreviation might be understood best by characterizing the sport situation as having a beginning, a middle, and an end. For instance when a ball is thrown it:

- leaves the thrower's hand;
- travels through space;
- arrives at your hand.

We have already discussed the fact that the catching response *must* begin *before* the ball arrives so that the catcher is on time to catch it. In fact the sooner the catcher can predict where and when the ball will arrive the more time he will have to plan and initiate the correct response. The more complex the movement the more time necessary for planning, selecting, and initiating it. It is to the performer's benefit, therefore, to establish or predict what will happen as early as possible. The ability to do this is called "cue abbreviation." Highly skilled performers can predict the end portion of a sport situation from a few cues that occur at the beginning. That is, highly skilled players can tell what will happen as soon as the ball leaves the pitcher's hand. They learn that certain occurrences or outcomes are associated with certain early cues. In addition some players "telegraph" their intent, their intended movements, and strategy long before they execute the movement. Then they wonder why their opponents always seem to know what they will do. Some players always stand a certain way when they hit a tennis ball to a certain spot; others may look at the place they intend to hit. Sometimes a player has a characteristic movement that "warns" the opponent of his intention. Defensive players, e.g., the tennis receiver, will try to figure out what offensive players, e.g., the tennis hitter, will do from early cues that will give away the intent. All players are doing the same, trying to figure out what the opponent will do, while preventing their opponents from determining what they will do.

Ability to predict what will occur early in a situation helps

The ability to predict what will occur early in the situation has positive aspects. The player who correctly predicts what will happen on the basis of early cues:

- can select the best response carefully rather than rushing selection and execution at the last minute;
- can shift attention to planning strategy for future responses;
- can get into the best position for execution;
- can prepare for the performance rather than being caught off balance;
- can feel in control of the situation because things appear to move slowly.

What is not clear is that there are also negative aspects of cue abbreviation if the opposing player is wise enough to use them. A performer who understands the tendency of players to respond on the basis of early cues can, for instance, hit a tennis forehand drive to the same place five shots in a row and then, on the 6th shot, he could do exactly the same preliminary moves but direct the shot to the other side. In all likelihood the opposing player will have predicted the same shot as the previous five and initiated a response to the same side. The player will rarely have time to recover and return the shot. What are some examples of this deception in basketball, tennis, soccer, or badminton? The ability to deceive an opponent in this way can sometimes make the difference between winning and losing.

Ordering of possible events helps performance

Probability planning. A final aspect which is somewhat related to cue abbreviation is the ability to determine the likelihood of events in the sport situation and order them from the most probable to least probable. How likely is it, for example, that a tennis opponent will hit a cross-court shot in response to a deep, forehand return? If a person hits a cross-court shot in that situation 9 out of 10 times, the probability is 90% that he or she will hit one the next time. If he or she only did that 2 out of 10 times, the probability that it will occur the next time is only 20%. In the first instance (90%) it would be wise to prepare for that outcome if the situation is conducive; in the second instance (20%) it would be unwise.

Most events that occur in sport are probabilistic. That is they occur a certain percent of the time under specific conditions. Knowing what these probabilities are enables the performer to reject some events as improbable and some events as most probable. This enables the player to prepare to execute certain responses in advance. When the offensive team finds itself in a 4th down and 10 yards to go in football, it will most likely punt but it depends upon where they are on the field. The defensive team will plan for the plays that are most likely while remaining flexible enough to respond if the opposition does something "improbable." The process of scouting the team that will be the opponent next week enables players and coaches to engage in a form of probability planning when setting up the practices for the week prior to the game. In basketball, coaches and players plan differently for different types of teams. In tennis you plan differently for different opponents.

Summary of input changes. It is helpful to think of the sport situation as an unfolding one in which one performer tries to predict what is going to happen before it actually does while the opponent tries to prevent him from predicting accurately. At some point a performer will be relatively certain what his opponent will do. If this is determined soon enough, through quick orienting, selective attention, probability planning, and cue abbreviation, there will be ample time to plan and initiate an appropriate response that will be successful in matching the created situation. If the focus is on the wrong portion of the environment, if attention is to the wrong cues, if the wrong event is predicted, or if the time taken to do any of these things is too long, the performance will be unsuccessful or selection and execution will be too late.

Teachers and coaches can help players to develop skill in all of these aspects by using the suggestions included in this section. These included providing verbal cues, manipulating probabilities, highlighting important cues, eliminating unimportant cues, or helping players prepare to perceive.

Players can help themselves by:

- forcing themselves to concentrate;
- practicing prediction even when not actually playing;
- trying to pick out the commonalities in different situations;

- being aware of the strategies opponents use in attempting to deceive you into making a mistake;
- watching better players;
- asking questions;
- trying to make your responses automatic so that attention can be freed to focus on what is happening in the playing environment.

DECISION-MAKING

The major factors related to improvement in the DECISION-MAKING segment of information processing are:

- *chunking* — the ability to see patterns of cues rather than individual cues;
- *schema* — the development of general rules to guide the planning and selection of movements to match the environmental demands;
- *automatization of movement* — the ability to execute movements without conscious attention;
- *intersensory integration* — the ability to integrate and analyze complex information.

Chunking helps simplify information processing

Chunking. The capacity for processing information is limited by the amount of information to be processed rather than by the capacity to process information. Beginners tend to process information one unit at a time while more advanced performers process information in sets of units. If a football player, for example, was unable to integrate the movements of the various offensive players into a single whole called a play their movements would have little meaning for action and the processing would take too long for the player to be of any defensive value. As skill level improves, sets of cues are seen rather than individual cues. The capacity for processing chunks of information is constant; the more pieces of information (cues) which can be handled in a single chunk the greater the total amount of information that will be processed. If, for example, you were asked to remember the following sequence of 0's and 1's it is unlikely that you would be able to do so: 001000011101111110001. If, however, you were familiar with a binary number system you could recode the 0's and 1's by sets of 3's where

000=0
001=1
010=2
011=3
100=4

101=5
110=6
111=7

and

001/000/011/101/111/110/001

would become

1 0 3 5 7 6 1

(a much simpler series to remember). What you have done is to chunk each set of three into a single cue. Instead of having to remember 21 digits you only need to remember 7, well within your capacity.

The cues in sport may be thought of as the 0's and 1's and the chunking as visualizing patterns of cues rather than single cues. In the same way the information load on the system can be reduced by chunking.

Practice should be in a variety of environmental conditions

Schema. A schema can be thought of as an abstraction based upon many instances of motor skill performance. The elements that are combined to create that abstraction are:

- the environmental conditions;
- the response and the result or outcome of that response.

In simpler terms it may be thought of as a *rule* which guides the motor response under changing environmental conditions so that it will always be successful. This rule is discovered by practicing under a variety of environmental conditions. After the rule is discovered the individual can then perform successfully under a wide variety of conditions even if he has never previously performed under those conditions.

Let us suppose that a ball is thrown at a target which is 10, 20, or 30 feet away. Through practice the following discovery is made.

Distance to target	Force of throw	Outcome
10′	1x	Success
20′	2x	Success
30′	3x	Success

The rule for the relationship between the distance to target and the force of throw is:

$$\text{force of throw} = \frac{\text{distance to target}}{10} \, (x)$$

To be successful the force of the throw must be the distance to the target divided by 10, times a quantity (x) which is constant. To throw a ball at a target which is 15 feet away substitute in the formula or rule and find that

$$\text{force of throw} = \frac{15'}{10}(x) \text{ or } 1.5x$$

Using this rule how much force would be used if the target was 25 feet away? Although schemas are more complicated than what is presented in the example the general idea of schema as a rule to guide motor performance in future situations of a similar nature is true.

Highly developed motor schemas enable a performer to select correct responses

As competency increases in a particular skill, such as the forehand drive in tennis, or the lay-up shot in basketball, the schema develops so that it is possible to quickly generate an appropriate response for a wide variety of situations. In a previous section we indicated that if in tennis there were three possible speeds, three possible directions, three possible spins, and three possible heights, the number of possible combinations would be 81 ($3 \times 3 \times 3 \times 3$). A highly developed schema would enable a performer to select or generate exactly the right movement to match the particular combination of speed, direction, spin, and height, quickly and easily. It would also enable the performer to account for differences in the starting position in planning the movement which will be successful. The concept is very important because it enables a performer to be adaptable and shortens the time it takes for him to make a decision about what he will do in response to particular environmental situations.

How?

Schema is developed by varying practice conditions

There are several factors that affect the formation of schema:

- variability of practice;
- availability of feedback about outcome and movement;
- intersensory integration.

The development of schema can be facilitated by varying the practice conditions. The teacher or coach should have the learner perform under a wide variety of environmental conditions. The conditions should be game-like and should represent a broad range of the actual possibilities. Feedback about the outcome and about the student's movement should be provided and/or the student's attention should be focused on outcome and movement feedback. The student should be helped to integrate outcome with movement and environmental conditions. Finally schema formation demands the ability to integrate information from the environment with information from the body, e.g., where the limbs are and where the body is, so that the resulting movement plan accounts for both the present state of the body *and* the environmental conditions (intersensory integration is critical to decision-making and will be referred to again later in this chapter).

What Else?

Automated executive plans and sub-routines enable the performer to devote more attention to game plan strategy

Automatization of movement. As skill level increases, the movement planning, coordination, and output phases become increasingly automated. This enables the performer to devote more attention to overall game plan and strategy because close monitoring of the movement phase is no longer necessary. A favorite analogy here is based on computer operation. Individuals refer to executive plans and sub-routines. An executive plan is an organizational process that controls the order and timing of a sequence of movements. A sub-routine is a standard movement sequence that is always executed in exactly the same way. It is performed without conscious attention. The executive plan by contrast is a flexible sequence of sub-routines consciously structured by the performer at each execution.

Well-practiced executive plans become sub-routines

Examples of sub-routines used in performing the forehand drive in tennis are:

- the grip;
- the ready position;
- the pivot;
- the backswing;
- the forward swing;
- the contact;
- the follow-through.

When appropriately executed in time and sequence, they make up the skill known as the forehand drive. It should be understood, however, that when the ready position was first learned it was an executive plan under conscious control and the sub-routines were the foot position, the body position, the knee position, the racket arm position, the non-racket arm position, etc. This executive plan became automated and no longer required conscious control. At that point the ready position became a sub-routine. In similar fashion each of the other sub-routines of the forehand drive were first executive plans and became automated, and so, sub-routines. Through participation in and practice of tennis, the sub-routines which make up the executive plan, forehand drive, will become less distinguishable and less and less attention to the individual portions of the forehand drive is required. When the execution of the forehand drive becomes automated the forehand drive becomes a sub-routine in the game of tennis along with the other sub-routines of backhand, lob, volley, cross-court, and serve. The automation of the strokes of tennis enables the performer to plan overall strategy and to concentrate on the total game rather than on each individual shot.

It is important to note that the action plans in the repertoire of movement sub-routines were executive plans that became fixed sequences through practice and experience. In addition these sub-routines are available for incorporation into other movement sequences. An individual who has had extensive past experience with racket games will be able to use the movement sub-routines in formulating executive plans for racquetball, squash, and other racket games and will not be starting from scratch in learning a racket game (in a similar manner some of the perceptual learnings will be useful, e.g., judging speed, direction, and spin of the ball).

Intersensory integration. It was noted previously that intersensory integration, the ability to judge the equivalence of input to different senses, is generally crucial to the operation of schema and to success at perceptual motor skills. A simple example would be to view a ball moving and to realize that the ringing sound you hear is related to that movement. To see a ball at arm's length and be able to reach out the precise distance and grab it or be able to close your fingers and pick up a pencil on the table are other examples.

Effective performance requires a notion of what is happening in the environment

Ability to recognize these equivalences is based upon practice at seeing and doing. Eye-hand coordination is based upon intersensory integration. You see an object and you reach the precise distance and grab it. Young children have difficulty accomplishing these tasks. With practice they will soon develop a visual-motor schema and capability to reach for objects. When children first learn to throw a ball toward a distant target they are not always accurate. With practice they soon develop the ability to precisely throw the ball the correct distance. They are able to do this because they receive feedback from the environment on each attempt regarding how far the ball traveled and its error in relation to the distance to the target. They keep attempting to throw to targets of different distances, sensing the amount of force used to throw, receiving feedback about the throw, analyzing the error, changing the plan, and repeating the steps. Eventually they form a schema such as the one described at the beginning of this section. This schema was based upon the integration of visual input and kinesthetic input (integration of information from two sensory systems), external information and internal information.

To perform effectively a player must have a notion of what is happening in the environment, on the tennis court, on the basketball court, *and* realize where he is in space, where his limbs are, and how he is positioned. To plan or select and execute a movement that will be successful in matching the environment, input from the body with respect to its position and its position in space must be considered.

OUTPUT

Controlling and integrating movement responses is a mark of skilled performance

The single most important change in the output segment is the ability to control movement execution. As players improve they are able to move their bodies as they plan. The movement they plan is the movement they execute. The force they want to impart to the ball is the force generated. Movements become integrated. Coordination of simultaneous body movements is possible. The player coordinates legs, arms, and breathing in the swimming stroke. The player can toss the ball and swing the tennis racket at the same time. Response execution does not have to be rushed; you are ready to execute the skill. Initiating the formulated response at precisely the right time is the primary problem.

FEEDBACK

Although there is a separate chapter on feedback, it is useful here to enumerate the changes that take place in the use of feedback as performers become more highly skilled. These changes are:

- advanced performers know what input to attend to in obtaining feedback;
- advanced performers can evaluate the cause and effect relationship between the response and the feedback;
- advanced performers can decide what adjustments are required in the response to correct the perceived errors;
- advanced performers can make the necessary corrections.

Self-directed learners analyze performance on the basis of feedback

The physical education teacher and coach can help the beginner become a self-directed learner who can analyze and correct performance on the basis of feedback by helping the learner attend to and evaluate available feedback. Some examples from tennis would be useful in illustrating an approach that might be taken.

The teacher might tell a beginning tennis player to observe the flight of the ball as it comes off the racket face and to remember whether the ball had a flat, high, or low trajectory. The teacher would then explain the relationship between the angle of the racket face and the resulting ball flight. The teacher might then point out the relationship between the racket grip or the looseness of the player's grip and the resulting angle of the racket face. Finally the teacher might point out how the player could adjust or change the grip to reduce the size of the error for the next attempt. The sequence of steps were:

- tell the learner what to look for;
- explain the cause (what I did) and effect (what happened to the ball) relationship;
- explain movement cause (grip) and effect (racket face position) relationship;
- explain how the movement error can be corrected;
- have the player try it again.

This sequence is elaborated in the section on feedback through the use of an analysis of error table.

Summary

We have seen in this chapter that important changes take place in the way input is processed, in the speed and efficiency of decision-making, in the control of output, and in the way feedback is utilized for performance improvement. These changes in information processing capabilities underlie the observable changes which take place as skill increases:

- performers learn where to look;
- performers learn what to look at;
- performers spend less time taking in information;
- performers learn to differentiate relevant (important) and irrelevant (unimportant) information;
- performers learn to predict the outcome from a few early cues;
- performers can discount (eliminate) certain outcomes as being improbable or less probable than others;
- performers begin to process "sets" or patterns of stimuli rather than individual stimuli;
- performers develop verbal labels for the patterns of stimuli that are characteristic of their sport;

- performers can integrate information from several important sources;
- performers have a highly developed notion of movements to match environmental events;
- performers can quickly select appropriate movements;
- performers can respond to novel events;
- performers can automatically execute movement segments;
- performers are capable of integrating the separate aspects of movement;
- performers are more adaptable, capable of successful performance under a wider variety of conditions;
- performers' attention shifts from the short range consideration of "this shot" to consideration of overall strategy for the long range aspect of "this game" or "this rally" or "this play";
- performers can guide their own learning through use of available feedback;
- performers can evaluate their own performance through use of internal systems.

Where Can I Find More Information?

Arnold, Ree, K. *Developing Sport Skills. (Monograph #2)*: Newtown, CT: Motor Skills: Theory into Practice, 1981.

Berlin, Pearl, et. al., eds. "Skill Learning and Performance." *Research Quarterly*, 43: 263-397.

Locke, Lawrence, ed. *Quest XVII: Learning models and the acquisition of motor skills*. NAPECW-NCPEAM, 1972.

Robb, Margaret. *The Dynamics of Motor Skill Acquisition*. Englewood Cliffs, NJ: Prentice-Hall, 1972.

Sage, George. *Introduction to Motor Behavior: A Neuropsychological Approach. 2nd edition*. Reading, MA: Addison-Wesley, 1977.

Singer, Robert N. *Motor Learning and Human Performance. 3rd edition*. New York: Macmillian, 1980.

Whiting, H.T.A. *Acquiring Ball Skill*. Philadelphia: Lea & Febiger, 1969.

Now, at last, the

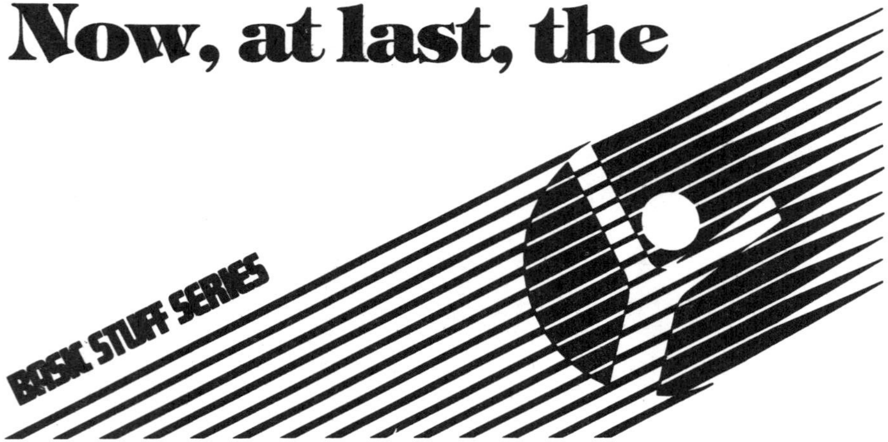

for K-12 physical educators . . .

Series I publications present the body of knowledge supporting physical education—order them now! Series II publications give examples of instructional activities to teach concepts—order now for April 1981 delivery.

Two exciting new series of publications provide teachers the BASIC STUFF to make physical education relevant to K-12 students.

Scholars and teachers . . . the experts in their fields . . . identify basic knowledge and present it in simple, concise language.

The new BASIC STUFF series will relate the knowledge of the field directly to the physical education class, providing the instructor with practical information and learning activities to truly physically educate today's students.

ORDER FORM—American Alliance for Health, Physical Education, Recreation and Dance

Title	Stock No.	Nonmember Price	Member Price	Quantity	Amount Due
Series I titles: Exercise Physiology	0-88314-024-1	$ 6.55	$ 5.90		
Kinesiology	0-88314-025-X	$ 6.55	$ 5.90		
Motor Learning	0-88314-026-8	$ 6.55	$ 5.90		
Psycho-Social Aspects of Physical Education	0-88314-027-6	$ 6.55	$ 5.90		
Humanities in Physical Education	0-88314-028-4	$ 6.55	$ 5.90		
Motor Development	0-88314-029-2	$ 6.55	$ 5.90		
SIX PACK (all 6 titles in Series I)	0-88314-031-4	$34.10	$30.65		
Series II titles: Early Childhood (ages 3-8)	0-88314-021-7	$ 6.55	$ 5.90		
Childhood (ages 9-12)	0-88314-022-5	$ 6.55	$ 5.90		
Adolescence (ages 13-18)	0-88314-023-3	$ 6.55	$ 5.90		
SET OF ALL 3 TITLES IN SERIES II	0-88314-030-6	$17.80	$16.00		
				Subtotal due	$
				Maryland Customers add 5% sales tax	$
				Shipping	$
				TOTAL DUE	$

Prices are subject to change without notice.

QUANTITY DISCOUNT — Deduct 5% for orders of 10 or more copies of a single title.

MEMBERSHIP DISCOUNT — Please note member price listed for discount, write your membership identification number here: ____________

Payment: (check one)

1. ☐ Check or money order enclosed. Please include shipping and handling charges as indicated in the chart below.

Less than $10.00	= $1.50	$50 - $99.99	= $5.00
$10 - $24.99	= $2.50	$100 or more	= 4% of total cost
$25 - $49.99	= $3.50		

2. ☐ Bill us (institutional orders only) PO # ____________ $50 minimum. Phone orders call: (703) 476-3481. Actual shipping and handling charges will be billed.

3. ☐ Charge to ($10 minimum): ☐ Visa ☐ MasterCard Phone orders call: (703) 476-3481. Actual shipping and handling charges will be billed.

Card No. ____________ Exp. date ____________

Signature ____________

Mail order to: American Alliance Publications, P.O. Box 704, Waldorf, MD 20601

Bill to ____________

Attention ____________

Address ____________

City, State, Zip ____________

Ship to ____________

Attention ____________

Address ____________

City, State, Zip ____________